Praise for *Essential Oils for Pregnancy, Birth and Babies*

"This book is a must have for individuals and families that want a concise, thorough and heartfelt reference guide to the life long use of essential oils for health and well being. Stephanie brings her extensive experience and her deep wisdom to this indispensable tool that will assist all people to achieve wellness, throughout the childbearing years and beyond."

—Jacquelyn I. Brenner, RN, midwife, CMT, JSJ and CST

"Finally, a concise but comprehensive book to assist you in using essential oils in all phases of pregnancy, labor, postpartum and babies. You will find this book to be an invaluable aid in guiding you naturally through a gentle birth experience."

—Billye Matthews, LM in Arizona

"I have just experienced prenatal, birth and postpartum care using Stephanie's recipes and protocols. What a difference! Since I am older now and have already had 3 children I prepared myself for a difficult pregnancy. Following her recommendations, I was able to function at a very high level up until the end. Birth was much more comfortable with her labor blend. Postpartum recovery is faster and I can see a big difference as I used her tips and tricks. You will be so glad you have this information either for yourself or so you can help others have an amazing experience during such a special time!"

—Roxane Bybee in California

"This book is powerful . . . beyond any I've seen pregnant or not!!! I love how well it has been put together, but most of all I'm impressed with the wellspring of usable, down to earth information it contains that is so user friendly!"

—Valerieann Giovanni, author of *The World of Mirrors* and artist

Essential Oils for Pregnancy, Birth, & Babies

Essential Oils

for Pregnancy, Birth & Babies

Second Edition

Stephanie Fritz LM, CPM
The Essential Midwife

Gently Born Publications
Sierra Vista, Arizona

Essential Oils for Pregnancy, Birth & Babies
Second Edition

Copyright © 2015 Stephanie Fritz

Cover Design: Whitney Horton and Imagine! Studios
Cover & Interior Illustration: Whitney Horton
Cover Photo: Lev Dolgatshjov/iStockPhoto.com

Interior Design: Imagine! Studios
www.ArtsImagine.com

The views and opinions in this book are provided to help educate the reader on essential oils and supplements for pregnancy, birth, and babies. It is sold with the understanding that the publisher and author are not liable for the misconception and misuse of the information provided. It is not provided to diagnose, prescribe, treat, cure, or prevent any disease. Pregnant or lactating women and people with known medical conditions should consult a physician as this information is in no way intended as a substitute for medical counseling.

Published by Gently Born Publications
Sierra Vista, Arizona

ISBN 13: 978-0-9855280-2-7
Library of Congress Control Number: 2015915423

Second Gently Born Publications printing: March 2016

Dedication

Thank you to my family, friends and clients who graciously allowed me to share their most intimate tender moments of birth! One of my greatest honors is serving you!

FDA Disclaimer:

The information, advice, statements, and testimonials made about the essential oils, blends, and products mentioned in this book have not been evaluated by the United States Food and Drug Administration (FDA). The information in this book and the products listed are not intended to diagnose, treat, cure or prevent disease, nor are they intended to replace proper medical help. It is always recommended to consult with a healthcare professional before starting any regimen with essential oils. User submitted testimonials are based on individual results and do not constitute a guarantee that you will achieve the same results—what works for one may not work for another.

My intention is to share the benefits of essentials oils to all. I provide as much information as possible about the oils and how they can be used specifically to pregnancy, birth and babies. Although I prefer a particular brand because it has worked well for me and my family, where you source your oils is up to you. Please use the information in this book to help you better understand how to effectively use them.

Contents

Introduction

*L*ittle did I know the first twenty years I worked with essential oils for personal health that I would find them extremely helpful in my midwifery practice. I often tell my clients, "If you get sick, there isn't much you can take while pregnant, but essential oils are very effective for most ailments and perfectly safe in pregnancy." Essential oils can be extremely beneficial during pregnancy, labor, birth, and even the postpartum period. I have found that using essential oils on a daily basis is the best way to eliminate a mom's emotional stress levels.

Substantial evidence reveals that a mother's physical and mental wellness during pregnancy can affect not only the outcome of her pregnancy but also her baby's well-being.

Over the years I have been honored to work with the most amazing families, providing them with a holistic approach to childbirth. We have worked together, each family and I as a team on their journey through pregnancy and birth. When they call me with an ailment for instance the occasional nausea in first trimester, I usually refer them to peppermint or cardamom essential oil, and they have done their part in following through on my recommendations, with good results.

You will read several testimonials from my clients of their personal experiences using these amazing oils throughout their pregnancies. Many of them have gone on to use them with their families as the main resources in their medicine cabinets. I feel gratitude for each one of these families for choosing this path, as it has made my job as a midwife so much easier. They are calling me less frequently (not that I mind their calls),

and they are empowered to take responsibility for their own health care instead of giving that responsibility to someone else.

In this book you will see specific recipes to address frequent complaints that occur naturally in pregnancy, but know that the two key words here are *common sense*. There really are no rights or wrongs when using these particular essential oils. I'll give you specific numbers because you want to know them, but really it's about using your intuition and common sense. Generally I say one drop for infants, one to two drops for children, and three to six drops for an adult, but that isn't always the case. Sometimes one drop for an adult is all that is needed. Everybody is different, and this is where your intuition comes into play. Don't be afraid to experiment. I will speak more about dilution and dosage recommendations in the next section.

I also frequently hear, "I wish you could be my midwife," and "I wish my midwife used these essential oils." My response to that is that if you can get your midwife on board, great, but if not, it's okay. You can use the protocols suggested in this book, whether your midwife uses essential oils or not. Again, you take control of your journey.

I will address this here as well as throughout the book: The brand of essential oils I use is one of the highest quality and purest in the world. I have not experienced any negative or adverse reaction to the essential oils I speak of when used in pregnancy. This is only my experience, but I cannot say this for all brands of essential oils. You will want to make sure that the brands you use are sourced from their native land; this is where the growing and harvesting conditions are optimal. This assures you that the oil has a high integrity and potency. The other thing to look for is that each batch is guaranteed to be third-party tested to assure you of its quality, purity, and potency.

The suggestions in this book come with lots of experience and much love, as I have enjoyed the journey with many moms and babies. I love the term "nine-in, nine-out"—nine months with babe inside your womb and nine months in your arms. This is the time frame I am focusing on.

Enjoy your journey, because this experience will only happen once for you, since each pregnancy is different.

What Is an Essential Oil?

*E*ssential oils are highly concentrated extracts that are naturally found in and distilled from different parts of a plant. This includes the leaves, flowers, twigs, the peel of fruit, bark, and roots.

A plant has oil sacks in these various parts, which protect it from disease. We can benefit from the same oils the plant uses to protect ourselves from disease. These oils can also clear out negative energy, promote a sense of calmness, lift a mood, and create powerful emotional responses.

Many essential oils have strong cleansing properties and are naturally antimicrobial. When used topically, their unique chemical structure allows them to pass directly through the skin for an immediate systemic response. Certain oils may be used internally to promote vitality and well-being as well as kill bacteria and viruses in the body. I love that I can use an essential oil to kill a virus, when an antibiotic can't touch it. This is because the virus lives inside the cell and most antibiotics can't penetrate the cell wall. An essential oil can because it is carbon based. Our bodies know exactly what to do with it.

Independently Tested Therapeutic Grade

*Y*ou may have come across many books that debate which, if any, essential oils are safe during pregnancy. Most of the time you will see a warning on the label or an advisory to contact your physician before using essential oils.

You may read that there are "studies" showing certain oils can cause spontaneous abortions, miscarriages, or uterine contractions. The problem with these studies is they are not clear on how pure the oils were, and how much they used. Certainly I can't imagine that any mother would agree to be a part of such a study using oils she thought would bring on complications or questionable outcomes in her pregnancy. Most of these studies were done with pregnant animals. These studies don't necessarily apply to human pregnancies.

Even with all the confusion surrounding the use of essential oils in pregnancy, I stand by my experience. I also stand behind the particular brand I use.

That being said, I have not been given stewardship over your body and your baby. Only you have this right, so if you feel there are certain oils that are not for your greatest and highest good, then by all means follow that intuition. I only speak from my experience.

You will want to find independently tested therapeutic essential oils from a reputable company that are 100 percent pure, naturally extracted from plants. Make sure they are tested in independent laboratories and do not contain fillers, chemicals, or artificial ingredients that would dilute their natural qualities. They must also be free of all contaminants, such as pesticides, herbicides, or any other chemical residues.

It's just as important to assure the presence of active compounds at optimal levels as it is to keep contaminants out of the oils. This is necessary to guarantee their safety and effectiveness. Many oils claim to be pure and therapeutic grade, but few companies actually apply the rigorous testing standards for chemical composition. All of the oils I use are independently tested therapeutic grade. They are sent to a third-party laboratory and tested using mass spectrometry and gas chromatography to ensure both the purity and the potency of each batch. They run these tests for one hundred forty minutes, ensuring that they will catch any and all compounds, both good and bad. Some companies claim to run these same tests, but the length of time is as important as the test itself. These are very costly tests, but this guarantees not only the purity of the essential oil but the potency as well.

Expecting mothers can diffuse, apply, or even ingest these pure-grade essential oils throughout their pregnancies to protect against common pregnancy discomforts: morning sickness, nausea, and even stretch marks. Essential oils can boost your immune system to help you have a healthy pregnancy.

The March 2, 1994, issue of *Nursing Times* published a research study titled "Using Aromatherapy in Childbirth." The study surveyed 500 women in the delivery room. Of these women, 74 percent used no form of pain relief except essential oils such as lavender, clary sage, peppermint, eucalyptus, chamomile, frankincense, rose, and lemon. The results? A high level of satisfaction was reported from both patient and midwife. The "aroma" covered unpleasant hospital smells and decreased anxiety among other patients and staff. In this study, lavender was seen to reduce maternal anxiety, provide pain relief, lighten the mood, and even calm contractions in early labor. Peppermint reduced nausea and vomiting, and clary sage helped to increase contractions.

Essential oils can be used throughout the entire pregnancy process. They can be applied to the bottoms of feet to enter the bloodstream within just a few seconds. Additionally, oils have specific qualities that act as a catalyst to healing and can be applied directly to the part of the body that they are best designed to assist. Essential oils can be applied topically, inhaled, or taken internally, as long as you are guaranteed they are independently tested therapeutic grade essential oils.

Methods of Using Essential Oils

*T*opically: Applying certain oils to the bottoms of your feet every day will help you stay healthy. Essential oils have been shown to destroy bacteria and viruses simultaneously while restoring homeostasis to the body. You may prefer diluting essential oils with fractionated coconut oil or another pure oil such as almond oil. You can use many certified pure essential oils therapeutically without dilution, but it is a good idea to keep a carrier oil handy in case of irritation. Diluting the oils will give you the same effect. However, carrier oils have larger molecules that slow down the absorption process. Diluting your essential oils may delay the effects, but the oils used will eventually provide the intended solution.

For massage, dilute fifteen to twenty drops of essential oil in one ounce of carrier oil. If the essential oil irritates the skin, dilute it with fractionated coconut oil, never with water. Water and oil do not mix, and water will actually drive the oil deeper into the tissues, which can increase the irritation.

Aromatic: Simply take the lid off and smell the oil, or use oils with a diffuser. As you inhale, the fragrance goes into the body through the nose and olfactory bulb and reaches the brain through the limbic system. You can also add a few drops to a spray bottle with distilled water, shake well, and spray into the air. Put a drop or two into your hand, rub together, cup your hands over your nose and mouth, and breathe in slowly.

Internally: The only essential oils I recommend ingesting are the highest grade of therapeutic essential oils. Please do your own research here. I have given you guidelines as to what to look for in a company or brand of essential oils. Add oils to drinking water, use them in food recipes, put them in gelatin capsules like any other supplement, or just drop directly under your tongue and chase with water. They are very concentrated. One drop of peppermint oil is equivalent to twenty-eight cups of peppermint tea.

General dilution ratio guidelines

- Mild oils dilute 1:1
- Sensitive oils dilute 1:2
- More caustic oils dilute 1:3

1:2 Ratio

- bergamot
- black pepper
- cedarwood
- eucalyptus
- geranium
- ginger
- lemongrass
- lime
- peppermint
- wintergreen

1:3 Ratio

- cassia
- cinnamon bark
- clove
- oregano
- thyme

General dosage guidelines

	Adult		Child	
	Ideal Amount	24 hr Max	Ideal Amount	24 hr Max
Aromatic	—	—	—	—
Internal	2–4 drops	12–24 drops	1–2 drops	3–12 drops
Topical	3–6 drops	12–36 drops	1–2 drops	3–12 drops

Categories of Essential Oils

I love the idea of categorizing oils. It makes using them so simple. Everybody is different, and there may be a particular oil that will work for one person but not another. Or a person may not like the smell of one oil but love another.

For instance, I am not a great fan of lavender to help me sleep, but I love the calming blend, this is a blend of lavender, sweet marjoram, Roman chamomile, ylang ylang, Hawaiian sandalwood essential oils and vanilla bean absolute. This blend calms the mind, relaxes the body, and soothes the soul, providing a safe haven from life's daily stressors. My husband loves the combination of equal parts of frankincense, bergamot, Roman chamomile, and vetiver. It helps him get a great night's sleep.

This is also good information to have as you are collecting your own medicine cabinet of essential oils. You may not have or want to use all of them, but, by using this method, you can pick another oil in that same category that works for you. Use your imagination and create your own blends of your favorite oils in the category of choice.

I will categorize many of these for you. As you get to know your oils and what works with your body, add your own favorites to the applicable category. This list is not complete by any means. It lays the foundation for you to start exploring and categorizing the oils you enjoy most.

Relaxation and Calming

- calming blend
- grounding blend
- bergamot
- clary sage
- frankincense
- geranium
- lavender
- patchouli
- Roman chamomile
- vetiver
- wild orange
- ylang ylang

Muscle and Pain Support

- massage blend
- soothing blend
- tension blend
- cypress
- frankincense

- lavender
- lemongrass
- marjoram
- peppermint
- Roman chamomile
- wintergreen
- white fir

Immune System Support
(Most essential oils are antibacterial.
I have listed a few of my favorites.)

- detoxification blend
- protective blend
- cassia
- cinnamon
- clove
- melaleuca
- Melissa
- oregano
- thyme
- rosemary

Digestive Health

- detoxification blend
- digestive blend
- cardamom
- fennel
- ginger
- grapefruit
- lemon
- lime
- peppermint

Skin Health

- anti-aging blend
- topical blend
- cedarwood
- frankincense
- geranium
- helichrysum
- lavender
- melaleuca

- myrrh
- rose
- sandalwood
- Roman chamomile

Fertility

*F*or many couples pregnancy comes easily, but others have a harder time conceiving. If you are one of those who struggles with this, it can be very stressful on both spouses as well as on the relationship. When you add up all the variables that have to be in perfect alignment for conception, it's a miracle anyone actually conceives.

Infertility is on the increase, and I believe this has much to do with our unhealthy diet. A zinc deficiency has been linked to infertility in both men and women.

A good diet of fish, dark leafy green vegetables, and nuts will help you increase your intake of zinc.

One question I am often asked is, "How can essential oils help with infertility?" Unfortunately, I think we have had a rise in fertility issues over the last couple of decades, and I feel much of it has to do with candida overgrowth in our gut. Cleaning up our diet and resolving the candida issue would help many women who are on the rollercoaster of infertility, and by rollercoaster, I don't mean a fun one. This often puts a strain on relationships and it definitely wreaks havoc on one's emotional state of well-being, sometimes to the point of depression.

When I talk about a candida cleanse, I often hear the response, "Well, I don't ever get yeast infections." You can have an overgrowth of candida/yeast, without ever getting a vaginal yeast infection. Candida lives in the gut. Other symptoms of candida might include:

- depression
- fatigue

- headache
- irritability
- poor memory
- PMS
- skin problems

Related, persistent digestive issues include:

- bloating
- constipation
- gas
- heartburn
- indigestion

Or you might experience other symptoms of candida overgrowth:

- coughs
- joint pain
- nasal congestion
- sinus infections
- sore throats

The list goes on and on.

Overall when you have an overgrowth of candida in your body, it definitely will weaken your immune system. A weakened immune system is the precursor for all major diseases. Yeast is a fungus and it feeds off a host, in this case, your body. It disrupts the endocrine system, and both your thyroid gland and ovaries are highly sensitive to yeast. Yeast is tricky. It mimics a lot of things trying to hide in the body.

To check for candida overgrowth, you can do your own saliva test. When you awake in the morning, before you put anything into your mouth, work up some saliva and spit it into a glass of water. After about fifteen to thirty minutes, look through the side of the glass. If there are strings coming down from your saliva, or if the water turned cloudy, or if your saliva sank to the bottom . . . you may have a yeast or candida concern.

So why am I talking so much about candida when you thought you were going to be gaining some insights on infertility? I believe if you take action in getting the candida under control, then most every-thing else should fall into place.

There definitely is another possibility: either low progesterone or an overabundance of estrogen.

I think more often it's an overabundance of estro-gen that causes the problem of infertility. We know yeast mimics estrogen, so when you have overgrown yeast or candida, your body thinks you have a high estrogen level. That leaves you with an imbalance of both progesterone and estrogen. Estrogen imbalance also results from the petrochemicals our bodies take in daily.

This is why I recommend cleaning up your envi-ronment and lifestyle as well as your diet. Are you washing all your fruits and veggies before eating them? I like to do this with lemon essential oil in a sink or bowl of water. Have you switched to a natural brand of hair products and skin care with all the good stuff and none of the bad? What kind of toothpaste are you using? What kind of lotions are you using on your body? Our skin is our largest organ, so anything we put on our skin is going directly into our bodies. What chemicals are you using to clean your toilets, sinks, and bathtub? These and many more questions are good to ask yourself as you pay attention to what your body is taking in.

Women's estrogen complex is an amazing product to help maintain a healthy balance of estrogen in your body. It goes in and eats up the bad estrogen to help balance out the good. We also have women's estrogen complex's partner, the bone complex. This combines bioavailable vitamins and minerals that promote bone health. It also contains vitamin D2 and D3 to help bones absorb calcium.

Women's estrogen complex can only do so much, but when you add the bone nutrient complex, you ramp everything up into high gear for the good in your body. These two products were created to be consumed together to help the other do its job better.

Thyme and oregano may help naturally increase progesterone. Both of these oils are in the GI cleansing formula I recommend as a cleanse when there is a fertility issue. Thyme is also included in the basic vitality supplements.

Stress plays an important role in this infertility topic as well. When our bodies are under stress, we produce the hormone cortisol. Its nickname is the stress hormone, and it inhibits our production of progesterone. Grapefruit essential oil helps prevent cortisol from blocking the production of progesterone.

Essential oils applied up the spine reduce the stress our bodies internalize. I love including this as a weekly treatment when spouses need their bodies to come into balance and readiness for conception. For this oil application, blend two to three drops of each: the grounding blend, lavender, melaleuca, protecting blend, massage blend, soothing blend, wild orange, and peppermint. This is also very beneficial throughout pregnancy.

Adrenal fatigue occurs after long periods of excessive stress and has a negative effect on all your hormones. Stress is a big factor in healthy or fatigued adrenal glands. Calming oils on your feet at night will help support adrenals. The oils below are also helpful when applied topically, directly over your adrenals. These oils will support them in all their work. The adrenals sit like little hats directly on top of each kidney located in the low back.

- 2 to 3 drops basil
- 2 to 3 drops rosemary
- 2 to 3 drops geranium
- 2 to 3 drops ylang ylang

If you don't have all of these, use what you have. I like to use two at a time and switch it up the next week.

Energy and Stamina complex may help with low adrenal function. This is a natural alternative to unhealthy energy drinks to support stamina and increase energy. Take as directed. Vitamin B5, pantothenic acid, is essential. No need to take extra; this is already in the basic vitality trio that contains all the vitamins and minerals your body needs in the optimal amounts.

Polycystic ovary syndrome (PCOS) is another common disorder than can disrupt fertility. *Poly* means *many*, so this is when there are many fluid-filled cysts on the ovaries. These cysts are not harmful, but they can be painful and cause irregular cycles, which can make it difficult to get pregnant. If you have PCOS, you may experience infrequent or prolonged menstrual periods, acne, excess hair growth, and have difficulty losing weight.

One of most successful treatments for PCOS is a healthy lifestyle of exercising, managing your stress, reducing your toxic load and a candida cleanse. A diet low in refined carbohydrates is important, because it helps regulate blood sugar levels. Losing weight is challenging with PCOS, but exercising every day and including the metabolic blend in your daily routine may also help regulate insulin and keep excess weight off.

Protocol for PCOS Support

- 5 drops frankincense
- 5 drops myrrh
- Mix the above in a gel cap and take 1 a day by mouth and insert 1 at night vaginally.
- geranium on the abdomen daily

Do this along with the recommended fertility protocol at the end of this chapter. Exercise daily and eliminate grains, or at the very least, go gluten free. This is a slow process, so you may need to continue for several months to see results. But be patient. It works.

Fibroid cysts are another common problem. Frankincense may help reduce existing cysts or prevent their formation.

- 2 to 3 drops frankincense under tongue morning and night

- grounding blend on feet morning and night
- geranium topically over the liver, adrenal glands, and/or the kidneys daily

Releasing/relieving stress is one of the most important things you can do when trying to conceive. I have found the following detox bath to be both helpful and relaxing during this time of cleansing and waiting. Baking soda helps to balance an overacidic system, and Epsom salt is helpful because the magnesium is absorbed through the skin and it is very calming. This is a great routine to do just before bed.

Detox Bath

- 10 to 15 drops lavender
- 8 to 10 drops geranium
- 1 cup baking soda
- 2 cups Epsom salt

I like to keep things simple, so I recommend the women's monthly blend every day. This relaxing blend contains essential oils that are often used to help calm feelings of stress and anxiety. It also helps to support and balance hormones. It provides temporary respite from cramps, hot flashes, and emotional swings. Some people can't wrap their heads around something that simple, so for those who feel they need more, here is another simple blend that you can rub on your abdomen daily for additional support.

Blend for Abdomen

- 10 drops clary sage (overall uterine tonic)
- 10 drops sweet fennel (may help reduce hormone fluctuation and help regulate menstrual cycle)
- 10 drops geranium (uterine and ovarian tonic, hormone balancing)
- 5 drops lavender (relaxes uterus)

Put the above in a ten milliliter roller bottle. Fill to top with fractionated coconut oil (FCO).

I have recommended this protocol to many who have struggled with infertility, with many positive stories coming back to me. I do a little happy dance with each story, because they committed to this hard work and were rewarded with a sweet baby bump. Keep in mind, this cleanup we are doing may take months to create the balance you are looking for. It's definitely not a "get rich (I mean pregnant) quick" plan. Be patient and know that you are serving your body well.

The metabolic blend, grapefruit, bergamot, and cassia, can help to kick down yeast and cut back the sugar cravings.

For men: the same cleanse as recommended for women, plus basil, clary sage, and sandalwood applied to the bottoms of your feet, your abdomen, and wrists.

The key is consistency in small amounts, allowing your body to adjust as it needs to.

Daily Fertility Protocol

- GI cleanse formula on days 1–10: Take 1 to 3 a day to cleanse the candida.
- Probiotic defense formula on days 11–15: Take 1 capsule, three times a day to feed your body the good bacteria and support your immune system.
- Detoxification complex: 2 a day to help nourish and detox body filters, liver, kidney, spleen.
- Detoxification gel caps: 2 a day to help open up the liver ducts so it doesn't become clogged with the cleansing you are about to do.
- Lemon essential oil in all your water to assist liver in its work.

- Basic vitality supplements: Take as directed to nourish your body with the perfect amount of vitamins, minerals, antioxidants, and omega 3s it needs.
- Women's estrogen complex: 1 a day to help eliminate bad estrogens in your body.
- Bone complex: 4 a day for bone and hormone support.
- Grapefruit essential oil: 10 to 15 drops under tongue or in veggie capsule once a day to help balance progesterone. You can split this up into a dose in the morning and another in the evening.
- Women's monthly blend: Apply to low abdomen, wrists, and back of neck to help balance hormones and mood swings.
- Avoid sugar, grains, dairy, fruit juice, and caffeine.
- Follow this protocol until pregnant, then discontinue GI cleansing complex and continue everything else.

Following is a list of essential oils recommended for fertility and progesterone. You don't need to use all of these; I just included them for reference as part of the fertility category. Any of these may be applied to bottoms of feet.

- monthly women's blend
- grounding blend
- clary sage
- cypress
- fennel
- frankincense
- geranium
- ginger
- lavender
- marjoram
- Melissa
- oregano
- Roman chamomile
- thyme
- ylang ylang

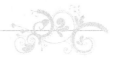

"Sharing my story of using Stephanie's protocol is my favorite thing to do! After a life-threatening miscarriage where I lost a tube from an ectopic pregnancy, I was told we probably wouldn't be able to conceive. I used Stephanie's protocol and we conceived the first month we tried. Now we have our little miracle-oil baby! Bless you, Stephanie, and all the amazing knowledge you share with us."

—Stacey

"About a year ago, I went through my first miscarriage. I somehow knew that with my age my body was not as healthy as it could have been. I thought it was my hormone levels that were off in some way. I was introduced to essential oils about a year later. I started on the Basic Vitality supplements, and about two months later I had a positive pregnancy test. I'm now waiting to have my beautiful little girl. I haven't had a baby in eight years, and I'm positive that the

essential oils and supplements I took helped my body hold onto this pregnancy."

—Catherine

"I didn't know about Stephanie or her book until the spring of 2013. I have PCOS and I've never had normal periods. I was told at nineteen I probably wouldn't be able to ever conceive without help. I was trying to get pregnant, but my thyroid was dysfunctional and I had bad reactions to the meds they prescribed. I've been using the oils for four years now, and so when my thyroid needed help, I started a protocol that I basically came up with on my own after doing research on which oils affect the endocrine system. After a month of following that protocol, my TSH levels were normal, and I had a normal period. Then I had normal periods for five months in a row! That has never happened in all my twenty-six years.

My fiancé and I found out we were pregnant!!! Such a huge surprise and absolute blessing!!! I followed Stephanie's book Essential Oils for Pregnancy, Birth, and Babies, *which was awesome. My four-month-old is strong and healthy and nearly off the growth charts!"*

—Patricia

"My husband and I don't have any children yet, and have been struggling with infertility for four years now! I have PCOS, and don't get a period or ovulate, making getting pregnant nearly impossible. My husband checks out healthy and good! We've been through all the fertility treatments, short of IVF, with no success. It's been almost two years since I had a period (my last one was brought on only by a prescription medication). Three weeks ago I started this fertility protocol, and almost immediately started heavy spotting and shedding! I am hopeful again, and very optimistic. Thank you!"

—Brandie

"My last baby I call my oil embryo because I used this protocol before, during, and after my pregnancy. A total life saver."

—Hilarie

"We are so excited because we used the oils and were able to get pregnant the first month we tried! A little background: We have two children, eleven and eight, then I was also a gestational surrogate for the family of a now-three-year-old and one-year-old twins. There were large gaps in between our natural pregnancies, and I never knew why. I got into the oils because of my chronic sinus infections. We started on the basic vitality supplements and found out about candida, the GI cleanse formula, and probiotic defense formula. Our whole family did the cleanse for six months. We still do it now about every two to three months. My husband and I noticed a huge difference in our bodies. I lost over thirty pounds, he lost twenty and continues to lose, and we are now both in a normal weight range for the first time in our adult lives!

He did some research and thought his testosterone was low, so he started to use sandalwood on his testis and geranium on his big toe. He felt a big difference in his energy and even saw more facial hair growth, which he was excited about. I was pumping at the time for NICU babies, and we decided I would stop so that we could try for another. I read Stephanie's book Essential Oils for Pregnancy, Birth, and Babies *and saw the fertility protocol. We had already been doing most of it except the women's estrogen complex and the women's monthly blend. I started implementing both of those into my daily routine. The day I stopped pumping, I started my first period! It was crazy that my body caught on so fast! My body was finally in tune and normal.*

We did not know how long it would take, but we were flabbergasted that we got pregnant the first month we tried! We are so thankful for the oils and the little baby growing inside me! This has been the best pregnancy I have EVER had, and I have used the oils as I normally do when not pregnant. I have even done the GI digestive cleanse while pregnant and not had any problems. Thank you, Stephanie, for giving me the confidence to use the oils while pregnant. When I was pregnant with the surrogate twins, I was a little scared to use the oils, but I will never have another pregnancy without using the oils throughout the entire term! Thank you!"

—Amy

"We had been trying for almost two years before I became pregnant with my third baby. As soon as I started Stephanie's infertility protocol, my cycles became normal and I became pregnant. I believe that the protocol in the book helped me conceive. Leading up to getting pregnant, I was using the oils on a daily basis. When I got pregnant, I continued using them because I felt I needed them, and I felt better."

—Anonymous

"Using the basic vitality supplements and the pregnancy and fertility protocols, I have been able to get my hormones back into balance post miscarriage and two chemical pregnancies. Through all of those experiences, I have decided on not having children. My *journey into honoring the female body and my cycle regardless of bearing children, I still follow the guidelines in* Essential Oils for Pregnancy, Birth, and Babies *because I find it to be the best way for me to be the most supportive to all aspects of my female cycle and body. I look forward to having these protocols help my hormones transition through menopause."*

—Namjeev

"I did the GI digestive cleanse and followed up with probiotic defense formula for three months in a row. I used the women's monthly blend over my abdomen daily. I took the full dose of the basic vitality supplements and one women's estrogen complex daily. I put rosemary and clove in a roller bottle and rubbed that over my kidneys/adrenals daily for adrenal fatigue support. I cleaned up my diet—virtually no sugar and ate as much whole food as possible. Mostly my advice to women in this situation is to be forgiving of your body and do some work to release any negative emotions that are present. I use lots of mood

management oils and citrus oils. I noticed they made me feel a lot better emotionally."

—Stacey

Nutrition

*N*utrition is an important element of a healthy pregnancy. Although this is a book primarily about using essential oils in pregnancy, I'm going to add a snippet of nutritional information here because I think nutrition is the key element to a healthy mom and babe.

I have everyday rules for moms to follow. The first one is protein, protein, and more protein! Oftentimes when your body is deficient in protein it will manifest that with edema. I recommend eighty to one hundred grams of protein every day as part of your diet. You can count your protein grams, but that can be a pain, and who wants to count calories or protein? I suggest you write down everything you eat for three or four days. Add up the protein, and this will give you a baseline of how close you are to the optimal amount.

If you are consuming close to eighty grams, Congratulations! You're doing awesome. However, if you're down around thirty or forty grams, you have some work to do. When you eat protein first thing in the morning and at every meal, with protein snacks in between meals, you are generally getting enough. When you add it up, you are consuming protein about six times a day. The metabolic protein shakes are a great way to get some quick extra, easy protein in your diet. I don't recommend it as meal replacement but rather a mid-day snack. Add some dark leafy greens to that, and three to four quarts of water a day with lemon essential oil in it, and you have a great diet for a healthy pregnancy.

I also recommend moms cut processed sugar and refined grains from their diet. If you can't remove them completely, at least cut down on all processed sugar and refined grains. A good rule of thumb is to cut out anything white. Candida thrives on sugar, and your body converts refined grains into sugars. This includes all fruit juices, dried fruit, soda, sweets, and ice cream. Even honey and agave should be avoided. It is best to eat fresh fruits and vegetables, and whole grains.

Sugar weakens the immune system. It weakens all tissues in your body, and it contributes to bleeding. This is where moms sometimes get a little defensive. They don't want to give up their sugar and white flour, but the benefits greatly outweigh this sacrifice.

The clients who have followed my no-sugar protocol have had minimal or no tears, very little blood loss, and much shorter labors than they previously experienced.

Many people ask if the metabolic blend is okay to use during pregnancy. And my answer is, "Yes!" It may help to regulate blood sugar, which can be an issue during this time. Its purpose is to stabilize your metabolic levels. It also helps with sugar cravings, and as you are committed to cutting processed sugar and refined grains, metabolic blend will be of great benefit to you. Just three or four drops three or four times a day will have a positive effect on your blood sugar levels and your sugar cravings. You can put this in your water, in a capsule, or just under your tongue and chase it with water.

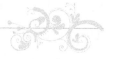

This was Bree's fourth baby, and she hemorrhaged with the last three. This time she wanted it to be different, so she agreed to give up all sugar. It wasn't easy, but she managed to be successful. When she delivered this baby, she only lost about a half cup of blood and didn't have any tearing. She couldn't have been more pleased, and said it was by far her easiest delivery and postpartum recovery. It's very common to have that annoying postpartum bleeding for four to six weeks after delivery, but when I returned for a follow-up with her on day five, she had no signs of any residual postpartum bleeding. It was like having

a regular period for five days and then completely stopping.

I have always recommended basic vitality supplements, or a whole food supplement as a prenatal vitamin, because your body can assimilate it like food. It knows exactly how to process it and where to distribute it in the body. I describe this as looking at a T-shirt with writing on it. If you look at it straight on, you can read it easily and know what it says, but if you read that same T-shirt in a mirror, your brain has to figure out what it means. It has to organize it and translate it from its mirror image before it is understandable. This is much like your body's organizing and translating of synthetic vitamins and minerals. Some of those ingredients are so foreign to the body, it doesn't know what to do with them, and so it just sends them to our body's elimination system.

I have discovered that since my clients have been using the basic vitality supplements, particularly the essential oil omega complex, the length of their early labor is often shorter. This is because the Braxton Hicks contractions late in pregnancy help to thin and ripen the cervix to make dilation more efficient. When women use omega fatty acid oils during pregnancy, these contractions will thin the cervix without causing dilation, therefore not promoting preterm labor. The baby's brain increases by weight four to five times in the last three months of pregnancy. Omega fatty acids are brain food for both Mom and baby. Essential oil omega complex also helps skin to be soft and supple, so if you are experiencing dry, itchy skin, more omega complex might be needed. It is not uncommon to double the regular dosage of essential oil omega complex.

Since I have been recommending basic vitality supplements, I have heard my clients say on a regular basis, "I have more energy." "I have more stamina." "I don't need as much sleep." "My back doesn't hurt like it used to." "I have fewer mood swings. My husband reminds me to take them because I'm more pleasant to be around." "I am more focused." "I'm less anxious." From my point of view, my clients are calling me less frequently with both physical and emotional issues

"I suffered with postpartum depression after my first baby. Stephanie suggested I take basic vitality supplements with my second. I used basic vitality supplements throughout my second pregnancy, and it made a huge difference in energy. I had no signs of depression. I had lots of energy, and I felt great."

—Ashley in Utah

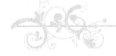

Basic vitality supplements, in my opinion, are the best prenatal vitamins you can take. Someone might ask about folate, whether there is enough in these vitamins for pregnancy. Most people don't know that folic acid (synthetic, in supplements) needs to be converted to 5-methyltetrahydrofolate (5-MTHF, aka methyl folate). Again, there is that conversion that the body has to do in order to assimilate it. There's a limit to how much folic acid your body can metabolize, and it plateaus at 400 mcg. If you supplement more than your body can process, you get un-metabolized, unusable folic acid floating around in your body, and it competes for transporting the good stuff. The basic vitality supplements have the perfect amount for your body, and your body metabolizes 100 percent of that amount. This also allows you to get the extra folate needed for pregnancy naturally in your diet. Since most processed food and all grains are fortified with folic acid, you should not have any problem getting the perfect amount needed for pregnancy. Natural folate is also found in those dark green leafy vegetables you should be eating every day. If you feel the need to supplement with extra folate, look for methyl folate 400 mcg from Amazon, iHerb, Vitacost, etc.

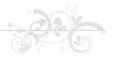

Darci was introduced to the basic vitality supplements with her seventh pregnancy. She was so excited to report at every appointment that her energy levels had never been better. She is a very busy mom with six other children, and she said she had more energy and stamina with this pregnancy than she had even when she was not pregnant.

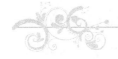

Another vital key to having an optimal pregnancy is getting enough enzymes. I recommend digestive enzyme complex to everyone, whether you are pregnant or not. This is a whole food enzyme, which helps many of your body's systems. The role of enzymes that we are most familiar with is their help with the digestion of proteins, fats, complex carbohydrates, sugars, and fibers. When taken with food, enzymes help your body break down these foods in the stomach so it can utilize the nutrients in the most efficient way possible.

They help your body to digest, absorb, and convert food into energy as well as help retain the nutrients in your body.

Often women experience heartburn or indigestion during pregnancy, especially in the third trimester. When they use enzymes in their diets, this uncomfortable symptom is greatly reduced. However, this is only half the story of enzymes. The other half we don't hear too much about. When you take enzymes on an empty stomach, they have many other benefits for your body. They actually rebuild and support connective tissue. Your connective tissue provides a structural framework for your body. Your whole body is made up of connective tissues: tendons, ligaments, cartilage, blood, bones, adipose tissue, and lymphatic tissue. Enzymes support and strengthen these tissues, which help to store energy and protect your organs.

Enzymes also help regulate thousands of other functions, including immunity, hormone regulation, cellular growth, and repair of organs, glands, and tissues. So, as you can see, enzymes are a vital part of our everyday routine.

GI Cleansing Formula and Probiotic Defense Formula

I don't recommend doing any cleanse with GI cleansing formula during pregnancy. I do, however, highly recommend the probiotic defense formula to help assist your body with its immune system. This is particularly important during the third trimester as your body is making colostrum. The probiotic defense formula aids in filling that colostrum with lots of good flora for your baby's stomach. It's that good flora that produces baby's vitamin K when it's first born.

Probiotic defense formula is part of my everyday routine for a healthy pregnancy. I recommend taking three per day the first five days of the month, and then continuing with one per day until the bottle is gone. Repeat this the following month and every month throughout your pregnancy and breastfeeding time. If you have to be on antibiotics at any time during your pregnancy or postpartum, I recommend increasing the probiotic formula to four to six a day for a couple of weeks to replenish and balance the good flora in your body.

Some women may experience excess yeast or candida, and wish to do a mild cleanse. The following digestive cleanse would be perfectly safe to do during pregnancy, followed by the probiotic defense formula.

Digestive Cleansing

- 3 drops melaleuca
- 3 drops lemon
- 3 drops thyme
- Put in a capsule once a day for ten days.
- Follow up with probiotic defense formula once a month during pregnancy to build

immunity that will be passed along to the baby.

- This is a milder form of cleanse. If you feel some sickness coming on, this is a blend you can safely take to address this.

Cleansing starts in the liver. It is easy to overwhelm the liver in the cleansing process. The liver is driven by nutrition, vitamins, minerals, enzymes and specifically fatty acids. The detoxification complex supplement is nutrition targeted to the needs of the liver as well as the other internal organs. The detoxification softgel is all about protecting the liver and open up the liver ducts so it can do its job more effectively. I recommend taking 1 to 2 softgels a day when extra support is needed.

First Trimester

*T*he journey into motherhood is an incredible and sometimes even overwhelming process, both physically and emotionally. While each mother-to-be is unique, there are some similarities among expectant women. Specifically, most women experience some discomfort during their pregnancies, brought on by dramatic hormonal changes.

There is a lot of discussion about essential oils and which are safe during pregnancy. Some even recommend avoiding certain oils during the first trimester that are acceptable in the second and third trimesters. I have used high quality therapeutic essential oils in my practice since 2008 and have never experienced any adverse reaction to any of them during any trimester or during labor and birth. I would not recommend just any brand from your supermarket in the same way. I would be cautious in choosing the highest quality of oils for use in pregnancy.

My recommendations are based on my experience with these oils, but I urge any person to use those two key words we talked about in the beginning: common sense. Trust your intuition, and if you don't feel comfortable with a certain oil, then by all means listen to that inner feeling. I can give a recommendation, but you are the one who has stewardship over your body and your baby, not me, so keep your power and don't give it away!

Breast Tenderness: This is often due to hormonal changes in the body. Women's monthly blend helps support balanced hormones, so it is my first go-to oil. You can roll it directly on the breast undiluted. The breast is a soft tissue, therefore it will go directly into that tissue immediately. Other oils that you may find relief with are grapefruit, lavender, and ylang ylang. You can apply these topically to breasts undiluted, or you may use a carrier oil if desired.

Constipation: Use digestive blend, lemon, peppermint, or fennel. Take one to three drops of each in water or in a capsule. Or you may massage the oil blend on your abdomen undiluted or with carrier oil if desired. You may use orange, cypress, or marjoram as well. Massage onto your lower back undiluted or with a carrier oil if desired. Other supplements that will be beneficial are bone complex and digestive enzymes.

Depression: The very best thing I could recommend to help bring you out of a depression is the basic vitality supplements. They are key to supporting your body through the many hormonal changes that happen during pregnancy. I have listed a few oils that support your body and work in conjunction with the supplements, such as invigorating blend, joyful blend, grounding blend, wild orange, ylang ylang, and frankincense. Diffuse any one or combine them. Experiment with your favorite blend of any two. For frankincense, place three to five drops under your tongue and chase with water or put in a capsule and swallow.

Edema/Swelling: I recommend drinking three or four quarts of water every day. You will notice when your water and protein are at the optimal recommended amount because you generally will not have an issue with excess edema and swelling. The following oils will help support your body in its circulation of excess fluid: invigorating blend, massage blend, cypress, lavender, ginger, and lemon. Mix three to five drops in a carrier oil and massage into legs, ankles, and feet. Add three to five drops of lemon to all your glasses of water.

Fatigue: I recommend invigorating blend, joyful blend, wild orange, lemon, grapefruit, and peppermint. Place one or two drops in the palm of your hand, rub your palms together, and inhale deeply for a quick pick-me-up. Massage onto back, shoulders, or back of neck, adding carrier oil if desired. The energy and stamina complex may also be helpful as an energy boost when feeling fatigued during pregnancy. Take as directed on the bottle.

Headaches or Dizziness: I use calming blend, lavender, peppermint, tension blend, or soothing blend. Apply to your temples, forehead, and the back of your neck, being cautious to avoid your eyes. Place a drop each of peppermint and lavender in the palm of your hand and inhale deeply.

Headache Blend

- 6 drops lemongrass,
- 6 drops marjoram
- 6 drops frankincense.
- Put in a capsule and take internally as needed.

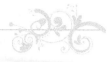

"When we found out we were pregnant with our first child, we asked Stephanie to be our midwife for our home birth. At the time we didn't know anything about essential oils. A few months into my pregnancy, I got a headache. Stephanie gave me some peppermint oil to try, and it worked wonderfully. I have been hooked on essential oils ever since."

—Sherri in Georgia

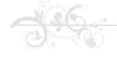

Heartburn: Try digestive blend, peppermint, ginger, and wild orange. Place one or two drops in a capsule or directly under your tongue and chase with water. Add one or two digestive enzymes to your meal.

Muscle Cramps: Cramps are usually caused by a deficiency of magnesium. Bone complex may help muscle cramps tremendously. You can also use marjoram, soothing blend, soothing blend rub, or massage blend. Massage onto affected area undiluted or use a carrier oil.

Nausea: Eat more protein at night, and your morning sickness will be lessened the next morning. It's all about giving your body the protein it needs. Most pregnant moms fall into the viscous cycle of being nauseated and not being able to eat or keep anything down, so if you can stay ahead from the beginning and eat twenty to thirty grams of protein before bed, you should notice a difference. The key is to eat enough; one boiled egg isn't going to be enough. The following oils may help ease the nauseous feeling so you are able to hold down food. Mix lavender, sandalwood, and ginger into fractionated coconut oil and massage into abdomen. Or even just apply a drop of cardamom behind your ears and on back of your neck. For some people, low enzymes may contribute to morning sickness. Increasing your enzymes to one or two on an empty stomach and one or two with each meal may help. Put three to five drops of fennel, ginger, or peppermint into a capsule and swallow. Mix one or two drops each of ginger and lemon in water with honey or stevia for nausea. Magnesium deficiency is also linked to severe nausea in pregnancy. Bone complex has extra magnesium in it. Sometimes a topical magnesium gel can be helpful as well. You get magnesium in the vitality trio, but some moms just need a little more to help combat that intense nausea.

Urinary Tract Infections (UTIs): Drinking three to four quarts of water a day is one of the key factors to avoiding a UTI, but if you feel a burning sensation during urination, a sign that one may be coming on, increase your vitamin C intake to 1000 milligrams every hour. Cassia is the best essential oil for a UTI. Put four drops each of cassia, oregano, protective blend, and thyme in a capsule and take every hour until you notice improvement. You may find it's better to take it with food, but that's not always the case, so try it both ways. Then continue to take three or four times a day for a week to make sure the infection is completely gone. Follow up with probiotic defense formula to provide good flora to your intestinal system.

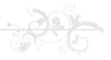

"Peppermint was a life saver for heartburn. I just put a drop under my tongue, and instantly the heartburn was gone."

— Ashley in Utah

"I used the peppermint in water for a refreshing drink throughout my pregnancy. When I felt gassy, it would feel like a stomachache. I used the digestive blend, and it worked like a charm. I would rub my tummy with the digestive blend and put a couple of drops under my tongue for bad indigestion."

— Christine in Arizona

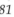

Final First Trimester Tips

Morning Sickness/Nausea Blend

- 10 drops peppermint
- 10 drops cardamom
- 30 drops lavender
- Mix in a five milliliter bottle and place few drops of this combo on hankie or hands and inhale deeply or apply to back of your neck and behind your ears.

Cardamom is the number one choice essential oil to help alleviate nausea. It blocks the receptor pathways of nausea. Apply to the back of your neck and behind your ears.

Peppermint is the number two choice. Simply diffuse in the air or put a drop in your hands and inhale.

Spearmint may also help with nausea and may even be effective for longer periods than peppermint.

Digestive blend or ginger is the number three choice to alleviate nausea. Inhale or put three to five drops in a capsule and swallow with water. Ginger is another oil that blocks the receptor pathways of nausea.

Mix invigorating blend in water to diffuse, or put a drop in hands and inhale.

Spray/Mist: Put twenty drops of peppermint, fifteen drops of lemon, and five drops of orange into four ounces of distilled water. Shake well and spray.

Second Trimester

The second trimester, like the first, brings on the pregnancy glow through the belly. You might have baby's first photo taken with an ultrasound to confirm that he/she's already adorable and whether it's a boy or a girl. Your baby's brain is developing, and around twenty-four to twenty-six weeks, your baby is beginning to grow rapidly. It's learning to breathe, listen, and kick, and your child may even respond to your voice.

This is the time when you will most likely feel your very best. Take advantage of feeling good: Go shopping, pamper yourself, and exercise. Swimming is one of the best exercises you can do in pregnancy. Make sure you are eating small snacks before exercise to boost your energy levels. Embrace the changes that are happening in your body.

This is the stage that you really start "showing," and this may bring a strain on your back. Using the muscle and pain relief oils can make a big difference in how you feel as your belly is growing.

This is also a great time to start massaging oils onto your belly to help support your tissues as they stretch. Some women are more prone to stretch marks than others, but using these essential oils through massage may help to reduce stretch marks and the discomfort that accompanies them.

Backache: Use soothing blend or rub lavender, marjoram, rosemary, wild orange, or massage blend. Massage any one or a combination of these oils with fractionated coconut oil. They can be applied undiluted, but for a massage fractionated coconut oil helps to cause less friction on the back.

Stretch Marks: Anti-aging blend is my favorite relief. You can use this undiluted or mixed with fractionated coconut oil for easier massage. Other oils that work well are a combination of lavender and myrrh, or any one of the following: invigorating blend, wild orange, cypress, or geranium, with fractionated coconut oil.

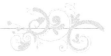

"I used frankincense, lavender, and fractionated coconut oil on my stomach for itching and to prevent stretch marks, and it worked! No new stretch marks, and it faded the old ones from my first pregnancy."

—Ashley in Utah

"Anti-aging blend is amazing on stretch marks! It was not available while I was pregnant, but I have used it on my stretch marks ever since it became available, and even on my old stretch marks it has made such a difference!"

—Jamie in Arizona

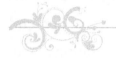

Final Second Trimester Tips

Stretch Mark Blend

Anti-aging blend is the perfect blend already distributed in a roll-on. You can use it undiluted or mixed with a couple drops of fractionated coconut oil for easier massage covering a large area.

- 10 drops cypress
- 5 drops geranium

- 10 drops invigorating blend
- 10 drops lavender
- 10 drops wild orange
- Add to base of six ounces of fractionated coconut oil.

Varicose Veins: Use lemon, coriander, cypress, geranium, marjoram, or helichrysum.

Apply directly to affected area. These oils may be applied undiluted, but you can use fractionated coconut oil if massage is desired.

Leg Cramps: Soak feet in a warm bath with five drops geranium, ten drops of lavender, and two drops cypress. Massage blend is a great oil to apply on legs at night. Sometimes a deficiency in magnesium and calcium can manifest in leg cramps. Try bone complex, a blend of vitamins and minerals that include vitamins C and D, calcium, magnesium, and other trace minerals that are all beneficial in preventing leg cramps.

"I was introduced to essential oils in my pregnancy. Since it was the time of winter that everyone seems to be sick with something, I right away fell in love with the protective blend essential oil. I rubbed in into the bottoms of my feet frequently to protect my body from the sicknesses that were going around. I never did get anything but maybe a day or two of a slight runny nose."

—Jenny in Arizona

Third Trimester

When you get to the third trimester, reality sets in. You really are going to have a baby. Incredibly, your baby will double in size during the last three months of your pregnancy, and in the last four weeks, your baby can put on even a half a pound a week. Your baby's brain is working overtime as it grows and develops. Your baby is beginning to prepare for life outside the womb. Your body and your baby are beginning to work together to get ready for labor and delivery.

The third trimester usually brings on the most complaints and discomfort. Most women experience fluid retention during the third trimester because body fluids double around twenty-eight weeks, so some puffiness is expected. For instance, you might not be able to wear your rings anymore. This is normal, but with a healthy diet and essential oils, you can keep this to a minimum.

Exercise: Swimming is a great exercise to do in the third trimester, because it supports all your ligaments and joints. You weigh one-tenth your body weight in water, so it's easy on your body. Swimming lengthens the chest muscles while shortening the back muscles. These are two areas moms complain about the most and ones that are often out of alignment as your body changes and baby grows.

Fetal Position: If you do find yourself with a baby that is not in the optimal fetal position, then peppermint or myrrh essential oil may help turn your baby. It is best to mix with fractionated coconut oil and massage from hip to hip in a rainbow motion up and around the top of the belly. For a posterior baby apply myrrh and peppermint on the low back in a circular motion to help persuade a babe to shift to optimal fetal position. Then crawl around on the floor for about fifteen minutes. Do this two or three times a day for optimal results. This may sound crazy, but you can also try having a conversation with your baby and asking if it's willing to change position to help you both during the birth. Spinningbabies.com is a great resource to help turn a breech baby.

Fluid Retention: This can become an issue, especially around twenty-eight weeks when your body's fluid levels double. The extra fluid puts more pressure on your body. Circulation is key to maintain a balance of fluid, and your body's circulatory system may be stressed and not working at its full capacity. There is a lot more in the body to circulate. Massage blend is great for circulation, and rubbing a little on your feet and ankles at night will be very beneficial. Along with circulation, sometimes a protein deficiency can lead to edema, or fluid retention. Increase your protein and water intake, put lemon in all your water, and massage any of the following on your feet and ankles: invigorating blend, massage blend, cypress, lavender, ginger, or lemon.

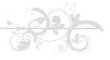

"Sometime in my third trimester, I started to retain water, and my ankles swelled up. At every prenatal Stephanie asked about swelling and, sure enough, you could not see my anklebones that day. She said I needed to increase my protein and have my husband massage some massage blend essential oil on my feet and ankles. I did as she asked, and never had another problem with swelling again."

—Kimberly in Arizona

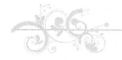

Edema Blend

- 10 drops cypress
- 5 drops ginger

- 5 drops lavender
- 5 drops lemon
- 10 drops massage blend
- Add to base of two ounces fractionated coconut oil and massage into legs, ankles, and feet. Or mix with a handful of sea salt for a relaxing bath.

Glucose Screening: Your doctor or midwife will generally do glucose screening test between twenty-four and twenty-eight weeks of pregnancy. This test checks for gestational diabetes. It may be done earlier if you have high glucose levels in your urine during your routine prenatal visits or if you have a high risk for diabetes. When you don't get enough protein in your diet your are more likely to spill protein in your urine and be at a higher risk for gestational diabetes, so get your eighty to one hundred grams of protein in everyday! This is a test where you must consume seventy-five grams of glucose followed by a blood draw. My recommendation to help insure you test negative for this is make sure you are getting enough protein everyday and cut grains and sugar from diet. The metabolic blend may help with cravings as well as help support healthy blood sugars. Basic vitality trio is also very helpful. The following blends may also offer support for healthy blood sugars in pregnancy if needed.

- Basic vitality trio
- 5 drops basil
- 3 drops coriander
- Put in capsule and take once a day.

OR

- Basic vitality trio
- 3 drops lemon
- 3 drops coriander
- 1 drop oregano
- Put in capsule and take two times a day.

Group B Strep: This is a bacterium commonly found in the intestinal track, throat, urinary tract, and vagina. Screening is usually done between thirty-five and thirty-seven weeks. The standard medical model of care if you are GBS positive is you will receive IV antibiotics in labor. As a midwife I must weigh in and include all the implications of GBS and then give my clients an alternative choice. I will not be giving you all the information here that you need to make that informed decision about your birthing, but I will give you an alternative approach if you do decide to go that route.

The basic principle and most natural approach is to provide Mom and babe's immune system with the support they need to combat any infection by building up the immune system. These are part of the everyday routine I have outlined in the beginning. If Mom has a healthy diet and is using the basic vitality supplements and oils throughout her pregnancy, she will be better equipped to deal with GBS or any other infection.

I feel bad when Mom has done everything right in her pregnancy—strengthening her immune system, populating her body with good flora to pass onto her baby—only to have that completely destroyed by using antibiotics during labor. There are, of course, times that

I might recommend the medical model, but those cases among my clients are few and far between.

I recommend to all my clients a chlorhexidine wash between thirty-six and thirty-seven weeks, then they repeat it once they go into labor. Chlorhexidine is an antiseptic wash that can eliminate GBS bacteria from the vagina. The benefits of this approach are that chlorhexidine does not cause the baby to become resistant to the normal colonization of skin and intestinal flora with healthy bacteria. If there are any risk factors such as chronic urinary tract infections, then I might recommend a round of essential oils in a capsule and on a tampon for a week.

Group B Strep Blend

- 4 drops lemon
- 4 drops melaleuca
- 4 drops oregano
- 4 drops protective blend

⁍ Take one capsule three times daily for one week, and in addition do the following.

Soak a tampon in:

⁍ 15 drops lemon
⁍ 15 drops melaleuca
⁍ 9 drops oregano
⁍ 1 teaspoon fractionated coconut oil
⁍ Insert into the vagina at night and remove in the morning. Repeat this for one week.

Nutrition: This is a time to sit up and take notice of your diet. This is also the time to cut the refined sugar and simple carbohydrates out of your diet, if you haven't already done so, and step up with your protein and dark green leafy vegetables and water. The normal discomforts of the third trimester will be minimal if you are following these guidelines from this point on.

Posture: Posture is another little secret that helps with an easier delivery. There are many studies that show posterior labors (when the baby is face up) are much more painful and complicated for both mom and babe. Most posterior babies often end up in C-sections, and a posterior baby born naturally can take longer due to how that fetal position affects labor. It's best to avoid a posterior baby from the beginning, and you can do this with your posture. Create an imaginary line going from your back straight through to your belly button, and make sure that line is pointing straight forward. For example, if you sit in a recliner lying back with your legs elevated, and that imaginary line points upward, that is not a good position. A better position would be sitting upright in a chair with your legs resting on a stool or something in front of the chair. Or sit on the floor in a tailor sit position which is sitting upright on the floor with your knees bent and your feet held together or crossed like Indian style and that imaginary line pointing straight forward again. Another good position is in a side lie on your bed. There again that imaginary line is pointing straight forward, as opposed to lying on your back with that line pointing straight up. For more information on this subject, Pauline Scott's *Sit Up and*

Take Notice! Positioning Yourself for a Better Birth offers more details and tips.

Pubic Bone Discomfort: This comes from your body releasing the hormone called relaxin to relax your pelvic joints so a baby can fit through the pelvis easily. It can be extremely painful and honestly delivery is the only thing that REALLY helps as it usually goes away after delivery. The homeopathic I recommend is Rhus Toxicodendron 30C from Boiron. You can find it at most health food stores or order it on Amazon. Your chiropractor can do a pubic bone adjustment to help with this discomfort and you can purchase a SI belt that is designed to compress and support the sacroiliac joints, thereby relieving stress and instability while supporting your hips.

Skin Problems: For acne or itchy skin, try Roman chamomile, geranium, lavender, and sandalwood. Some women experience the mask of pregnancy. This is a brownish skin pigmentation that usually diminishes after pregnancy, but you can use the anti-aging blend to help diminish this temporary change in pigment during pregnancy. Some moms develop a rash during pregnancy that is accompanied by intense itching; some might refer to this as PUPPP (short for pruritic urticarial papules and plaques of pregnancy). This is the most common skin rash pregnant women experience. It often occurs around thirty-three weeks, but it can present itself anytime during pregnancy. A blend of equal parts of frankincense, helichrysum, and lavender mixed with fractionated coconut oil may help this condition. Apply to rash for instant support two to three times a day. The body has four natural elimination channels; GI track, kidneys, lungs and skin, so when you develop skin irritations or rashes, you may want to consider giving the liver a little more support. The detoxification complex is nutrition targeted to the needs of the liver as well as the other internal organs. The detoxification softgel is all about protecting the liver and opens up the liver ducts so it can do its job more effectively. I recommend taking 1 to 2 softgels a day during pregnancy or breastfeeding when extra support is needed.

Sore Muscles: Mix any of the following with fractionated coconut oil and massage into sore muscle area: soothing blend, lavender, ginger, marjoram, wintergreen, tension blend, or massage blend. You might also find the soothing blend complex helpful with sore muscles and low back pain.

Sleep: To enhance your sleep, try calming blend or lavender on the bottoms of your feet at night or diffused. One of my favorite blends to help with relaxation at night is equal parts bergamot, Roman chamomile, and frankincense. This can be applied to the bottoms of your feet or around your neck. You can even try a drop or two of each in the diffuser. Another favorite blend for sleep is equal parts of calming blend, grounding blend, and either vetiver or juniper berry.

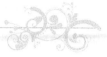

"I used lavender to help me get a good night's sleep in that last month of pregnancy."

—Jenny in Arizona

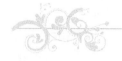

Perineum Massage: This is an old practice that has some debate around it. Some moms and midwives swear by it, and others are opposed. I will give you some direction here, and you can see if it feels right for you. My experience has been that it doesn't matter whether you massage or not. Just using a spray or drops of oil on your perineum will make a difference.

Perineum massage is meant to help to your body get ready for baby to be born. It's much like stretching a balloon before blowing it up. This helps to increase elasticity of the perineum, allowing for baby to fit through with minimal stress or tearing in that area.

Mix any of the following with fractionated coconut oil: Roman chamomile, geranium, sandalwood, or frankincense. Using clean hands, put your thumb (or have your partner do this) about one to one and a half inches inside your vagina. Press gently but firmly downward toward your rectum. You may feel a little discomfort, or maybe even tingling. A little discomfort is fine, but burning is not. These tissues are extremely sensitive, and may even be a little swollen, and with too much pressure you could cause bruising. Keeping a steady pressure, move fingers or thumb from side to side and back and forth along both sides in a U-shaped motion on the lower half of the vagina. Continue this for three to five minutes. This can be repeated daily with gradually increasing pressure and time. After about a week, you will notice an increase in stretchiness in that area.

Jan had an episiotomy with her first baby. When her second one came along, she had a pretty significant tear along her previous episiotomy line. This was her greatest fear with baby number three. In fact, her body never completely recovered from her first two deliveries. She would come to her prenatal appointment with a heavy heart and immeasurable fear. We talked about her past experience at length and decided to try frankincense and helichrysum everyday as a peri spray to heal and repair those tissues as well as prepare for her next delivery. She agreed and was very committed. She had an incredible birth without a tear! She couldn't have been any happier. When baby number four came around, she applied anti-aging blend every day to that area. Again she had no tear. It was by far her easiest pregnancy and recovery because she knew her body would respond to the oils.

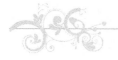

Hemorrhoids, Varicose Veins, and Constipation: These are related, but in pregnancy constipation is usually the cause for the other two. A diet high in fiber with plenty of water will usually help the constipation issue. In pregnancy blood circulation is often more concentrated in the upper body, and this is another reason for swelling in feet and ankles. Varicose veins usually are from the weight of the uterus pressing on the pelvic and leg veins and weakening them. A blend of geranium, cypress, and lavender mixed with fractionated coconut oil may help both alleviate and prevent the discomfort of hemorrhoids. Apply directly on area affected and massage gently.

Hemorrhoid Blend

- 4 drops cypress
- 4 drops helichrysum
- 2 drops peppermint
- 2 tablespoons fractionated coconut oil or witch hazel

Labor and Birth

*T*his is the event you have waited for. There's no changing your mind now. Your body and this baby have come into perfect alignment with each other, and this is the day. Labor is hard work. Some might interpret that as painful, and some may describe it as intense. Either way, there is a lot going on in your body on all levels: emotionally, physically, mentally, and spiritually. One of the things I love about essential oils is how they address the body on all these levels. The body is a symphony, and when one of these areas is out of balance, it can throw the whole body out of tune.

You may want to dilute essential oils used in labor with fractionated coconut oil, not because they can't be used undiluted, but because usually they accompany a massage, and massage just feels better with a carrier oil. Some moms may be very sensitive to smells while in labor, as some scents can be very overwhelming, so remember that a little goes a long way.

Geranium enhances circulation and is good for labor management techniques, which focus on breathing and pain relief. The massage blend is also a great choice to improve circulation and relaxation, and it is soothing to both mind and body. The back and shoulders are often areas of tension; massage with fractionated coconut oil to these areas for relief of stress and tension.

Basil can be used to relieve pain during labor and in turn gives you the strength needed to endure with greater ease. Moms can usually cope with labor contractions until they begin to be too painful. When they aren't able to manage the pain any longer, labor becomes difficult. Have your husband massage basil with fractionated coconut oil on your low back.

Black pepper is similar to basil and can be used to relieve pain in labor. This can be especially helpful if you experience back labor. Have your husband massage black pepper onto your lower back with fractionated coconut oil.

Calming blend is designed to reduce stress by calming the nervous system, creating a sense of well-being, and improving health through the natural reduction of stress and its related symptoms. It also encourages a loving relationship between Mom, Dad, and the new babe, bringing them into balance with a sense of wholeness.

Grounding blend is the perfect blend to balance and ground you. It can be applied on the feet to help relax you and increase a sense of courage as you go through the birthing process. It helps balance electrical energies in the body, giving feelings of courage, confidence, and strength. This blend is empowering.

Grounding blend may help the body self-correct its balance and alignment of the spine. It may help overcome fear during the labor process. It brings a feeling of calmness, peace, and relaxation. Grounding blend helps to ground and connect you with your lower body. Oftentimes moms want to run away from contractions and the sensations going on in that part of their bodies. This can come from a past experience, and those same sensations are bringing up difficult memories (such as trauma of some sort). Grounding blend helps Mom to stay present and stable in the moment and focus on what her body is doing. It gives her an inner feeling of courage and strength and a feeling of "I can do this."

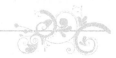

I was at Gabby's birth, and I knew there had been some abuse in her past, so I put grounding blend on my neck and heart area to keep me 100 percent present and aware of her needs. We were sitting together. I was rubbing her back. She was swaying side to side, leaning into me each time she swayed my way. I soon realized she was lingering longer as

she swayed my way and taking in the aroma of my neck. I just smiled. I knew this was helping her stay grounded as well. Later when she was in the birth tub, she said, "There was some smell I was smelling on you. Can I smell that again?" I knew what she was referring to, so I went to my bag of oils and got out the grounding blend. This was when I first started using essential oils at birth, and I was still learning my comfort level in using them in labor with clients, so I just opened the bottle and allowed her to smell it. She continued to sway in the tub, and with every sway my direction, she took a big whiff of grounding blend directly from the bottle. After the birth we visited on the phone. She commented that she needed that oil blend in her everyday life. It was so powerful for her during her birth; it was that aroma that kept her present. She said prior to my opening the bottle when she was in the tub, she was having flashbacks of her past, but when she smelled it, she could stay in the present moment. I realized in that moment how powerful grounding blend was and the difference it made for this mom. I now use grounding blend at EVERY birth, and I'm not afraid to apply it directly on Mom undiluted, or I even put a few drops in her birth tub.

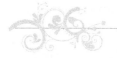

Clary sage is a uterine tonic that assists with effective contractions. It may help strengthen contractions once they have started. It doesn't bring on contractions unless everything is already in alignment for labor. Once labor has started, you can apply a drop topically to your pinky toes at the nail bed, the inside ankle bones on both feet, and on the low abdomen every fifteen to twenty minutes or until the strength of contractions has increased. I don't recommend doing this until labor has started or after forty weeks. It can be euphoric and wonderful for relieving anxiety as well. It calms the nervous system, relieves tension, strengthens labor, and helps with expelling afterbirth. I recommend blending clary sage with essential oils like geranium and lavender.

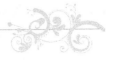

"I used clary sage for my contractions, and I felt it helped make each contraction more effective and come on stronger and faster!"

—Phalecia in Utah

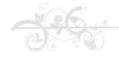

Invigorating blend is a combination of all the citrus oils. It makes an excellent delivery room diffuser blend. Not only are the citrus oils naturally antibacterial, they are antidepressant, refreshing, and provide for an overall positive disposition.

Joyful blend is great for creating a joyful experience. It is uplifting and calming. Joyful blend is a blend of oils that help balance and stabilize emotions. It gives Mom feelings of transformation. Lots of big changes in her life are about to happen, and labor can be overwhelming. Often in labor a mom will get caught up with those feelings of being overwhelmed by what's to come, and those feelings can stall the labor's progression. Joyful blend raises her energy levels on a physical as well as an emotional level.

Lavender is best for delivery room atmosphere. Lavender is very calming and soothing and can bring a spirit of gentleness to the delivery room. Grounding blend and wild orange are also a great combination for the delivery room.

"I work with Stephanie in her midwifery practice and learned about using essential oils during pregnancy, labor, and birth. While I was in Haiti on a mission trip providing midwifery services, in the early hours of the morning a first-time young mother and husband HYSTERICALLY came to the birthing center in labor. She kept saying over and over in French, "Je suis cassé," which means, "I am broken." I checked her vital signs. They were slightly elevated but still within normal range, and the baby sounded well. Her water had not broken, and she was three to four centimeters dilated. Since there is very little

childbirth education in Haiti, it was obvious that this couple did not know what to do and just needed some encouragement and rest. I put some lavender on the mama's foot, and within thirty minutes, both she and her husband were in a deep, deep sleep. Contractions would wake her up from time to time, but then she would go back to snoring! After a good night's sleep and a calmer approach, she was ready to give birth to a healthy baby."

—Misty in Arizona

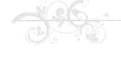

Myrrh may help to intensify contractions. It will not bring contractions on, but combined with clary sage it may help strengthen them. This is a great combo for stalled labor.

Peppermint, when inhaled, can help reduce anxiety and hypertension. On the lower back, it can be cooling. Peppermint may help to turn a breech baby. Apply with fractionated coconut oil to the belly and gently massage. Myrrh can also be added to assist with repositioning baby.

Labor Support Blend

Diffuse grounding blend and wild orange, which you can also apply topically on the bottoms of feet, the back of the neck, and the ears.

Recipe Once Labor Has Started

- 15 drops carrier oil
- 5 drops ylang ylang
- 5 drops helichrysum
- 5 drops digestive blend
- 2 drops peppermint
- 2 drops clary sage

- Massage on the insides of ankles, the lower stomach, and the lower back to relieve nausea and muscle pain.

Grounding and Calming Spray

- 40 drops grounding blend
- 4 ounces distilled water in a glass spray bottle

Relax and Focus Diffuser Blend

- equal parts of wild orange and peppermint

Relaxing Blend

- 4 to 5 drops Roman chamomile
- 2 to 3 drops frankincense
- 2 to 3 drops bergamot

   ➣   apply to bottoms of feet

Perineum Support while Pushing

Helichrysum is my oil of choice, to create lubricant oil for crowning. Mix twenty drops with four tablespoons of fractionated coconut oil and apply all over perineum area. This helps to stretch tissue while minimizing discomfort and swelling, and it helps avoid occasional tears. It also may help prevent bruising of baby's head. I like to call helichrysum the arnica of essential oils. Arnica is a homeopathic that helps with bruising, bleeding, and trauma. These are all the qualities of helichrysum too.

Perineum Support for Pushing Stage

   ➣   4 tablespoons fractionated coconut oil
   ➣   20 drops helichrysum

- 20 drops frankincense
- Gently massage on the perineum during crowning and birth of baby's head for the occasional bruising, swelling, and bleeding.

"Our son, Micah David, was born around the beginning of December. Stephanie used essential oils on me during the labor and birth of our son, and I know they made a difference. She used helichrysum on my perineum as he was crowning to help me to stretch, minimizing the chance of tearing. Now when I smell helichrysum I'm taken back to that amazing moment our son entered this world!"

—Jenny in Arizona

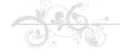

Cesarean Section

You can use the same oils for a c-sec as you would with a vaginal birth. Grounding blend and wild orange are great to diffuse to support a calm feeling when go in for your c-sec. I would recommend putting a drop or two of each in your hands and inhaling deeply then applying to back of neck and around your ears. The relaxing blend listed above might be beneficial as well.

Gemstones with their powerful energies and profound relationship with the human body are the perfect energy medicine tools. Like other forms of energy medicine, gemstone energy medicine uses the body's natural healing gifts to nourish and heal us in multiple ways. Each type of gemstone has a unique energy that can focus and amplify this healing force and produce specific therapeutic effects. Along with essential oils, therapeutic gemstones are part of my natural pharmacy that I use every day for personal use as well as with my clients. Wearing a gemstone necklace can energize and inspire us, help restore our health, and initiate enduring changes.

Just like the essential oils, the quality and purity and potency must be the very best there is. The gems in a therapeutic necklace must be high enough in quality to deliver the healing and transformation we seek from them. If a gemstone's inherent quality is insufficient, if it is filled with impurities and flaws and its color is muddy, its energy will be distorted and weakened. The dyeing, irradiation, and waxing that gems are commonly subjected to in the jewelry industry also corrupt the gemstones' healing energies.

I personally use ALL of these therapeutic gemstone necklaces. If you see me in person, I ALWAYS have a gemstone necklace on, just like I ALWAYS have essential oils on.

Two I have in my birth bag are:

- **Riverstone:** Helps Mom with labor and gives her the confidence and encouragement to push her through transition with grace and ease.

    Poppy Jasper: Helps give Mom energy needed to push baby out. It's like an extra boost of when you think you can't go on another minute.

There are too many other helpful gemstones to name here, so please visit gemisphere.com to learn more about these amazing tools. When you mention I directed you to their site, they will offer you 15% off your first order. Use code FRITZ15.

Postpartum

I like to call postpartum the "babymoon." This is a time to bond with this little bundle of love and be pampered yourself. Babies change your world. Enjoy this sacred time, because your experience with this baby will only happen once for you. There is still a lot going on in your body. It has just been though a BIG event, and it needs time to recover and come back into a new balance. This is an exciting time, but it is also one of many changes, both hormonal and physical. Give your body the space it needs to come back into its perfect homeostasis.

After the newness of the baby's arrival wears off, everyone's life goes back to the way it was before the birth, except for yours. Dad goes back to work, siblings go back to school, and no more meals are brought in, if you were lucky enough to have them. You and your body are taking care of two people now, and your body is doing some major changes.

Day four of this babymoon period is usually the hardest, so my best advice is rent a chick flick, one that will surely make you cry. This will give you a way of releasing your feelings of being overwhelmed in a way that is normal to others, so you don't have to explain them, because you wouldn't be able to if you tried. This is a hormonal change that causes unexplained emotions, even if you're not normally an emotional person. Usually all you need is a good cry, and the next day is generally better. Grounding blend will be your friend, so use it every day on the bottoms of your feet, the back of your neck, and even on the bottoms of your baby's feet. Dads, this is a GREAT day for you to break out your massage skills and pamper Mom with TLC. Applying essential oils to her back would be a perfect way to help her relax and release tension and feelings of being overwhelmed. The essential oils I recommend is two to three drops of grounding blend, lavender, melaleuca, protecting blend, massage blend, soothing blend, wild orange, or peppermint.

Afterpains are inevitable. Your uterus has grown over the last nine months almost twenty-five times its normal size. Your body contracts after birth to help it return to its pre-pregnancy size. This usually takes anywhere from four to six weeks. When you experience afterpains (menstrual-like cramps), your uterus is contracting and clamping down like a tourniquet on all those blood vessels that fed your baby through the placenta. This is its job so you don't continue to bleed, but these cramps can be very intense, and even though it is your body doing what it should be doing, it is very uncomfortable.

These afterpains continue for two to three days. They are worse when you breastfeed, because your body is responding to the oxytocin hormone released when breastfeeding. Oils that help with this discomfort are lavender and white fir. Apply directly to low abdomen undiluted for instant relief. The reason for choosing these particular oils is because your uterus is a muscle, and it's contracting. Think about the oils in the muscle category. Any of those oils would work, but lavender and white fir are both very gentle oils, so if baby happens to touch your belly, those oils won't be too harsh for baby's tender skin. This can be helpful after a cesarean section also.

Women's monthly blend is a women's hormonal blend that is also very effective and gentle to baby's skin. This blend helps to balance emotions as it releases tension from the uterus.

Urinating can be an issue, as some moms may have swelling after birth, and this makes it difficult to urinate. A drop of peppermint in the toilet helps with this. Often a little smell of grounding blend, lavender, or calming blend will help with the relaxation your body needs to let go.

For **peri spray**, use anti-aging blend, twenty to thirty drops, and fill the rest of your spray bottle with fractionated coconut oil. This peri spray may be used on a circumcision also, as it is very soothing and helps with the healing process.

Anti-aging blend was created specifically for skin and longevity, and it was named appropriately, but this oil has countless other benefits. It is one of my favorite blends because of the amazing oils that make up this blend. It can actually accelerate tissue repair, and so it has become my favorite oil of choice for soothing and healing the tender perineum areas after childbirth. If you don't have anti-aging blend, frankincense and lavender are a good mix for the same area.

Postpartum Blend

- ✍ 10 drops frankincense
- ✍ 10 drops lavender
- ✍ Combine these in a fifteen-milliliter bottle with a spray top. Fill almost to the top with distilled water. Use this to spray on the perineum after birth to soothe and heal during postpartum time. Moms who have their babes circumcised have used this same spray on the circumcised area. They know from personal experience how soothing it feels.

Grounding blend helps your body find a new balance. Use every day on the bottoms of your feet. This is a blend that is especially helpful to keep you in the present moment and you focus on everyday tasks. Grounding blend is made up of tree oils. Trees have roots that are planted firmly into the earth, so that tree can withstand the storms that come and not topple over. Grounding blend brings those same benefits into our lives. It keeps us grounded and connected to the earth's energy and in the present moment, so when life's stresses come as your body recovers on all levels, you can stand firm and not topple over.

What new mom doesn't need some **rest and relaxation time**, whether it's her first babe or her sixth? That peaceful, calm feeling is vital for successful breast-feeding. The following is a blend that is great to use aromatically. Mix geranium, lavender, sandalwood, ylang ylang, two or three drops of each, in the diffuser.

Caesarean moms, digestive blend may help gas pains that occasionally come after anesthesia. Even if those gas pains are in your shoulder, just apply topically to area of concern. Anti-aging blend may be especially helpful postpartum for your incision. Use it everyday morning and night on your scar after staples or tape has been removed. This is already the perfect blend to help the appearance of fine lines and scars. It also has helichrysum in it, which is beneficial for tissue repair.

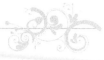

"After a very intense delivery at home, I used a mixture of frankincense and lavender for help in my own healing. We also used frankincense and myrrh with our baby. Since then, I have continued to research and use essential oils for our growing family's needs."

—Sherri in Georgia

"I really liked the peri spray Stephanie made for me of lavender and frankincense. It was very soothing and I think it increased my healing."

—Ashley in Utah

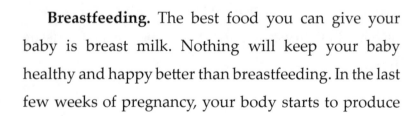

Breastfeeding. The best food you can give your baby is breast milk. Nothing will keep your baby healthy and happy better than breastfeeding. In the last few weeks of pregnancy, your body starts to produce colostrum. It is high in carbohydrates and protein but low in fat. It's exceptionally high in antibodies to help keep your baby healthy. It's the easiest food for your baby to digest, which makes it the perfect food for your baby's first feeding. It also contains high concentrations of leukocytes, which are protective white cells that destroy bacteria and viruses. The probiotic defense formula you have been taking throughout your pregnancy adds good bacteria and good flora to your colostrum, so those benefits are passed to your baby as you breastfeed. This helps to populate your baby's digestive tract with good bacteria that destroy disease.

Colostrum is measured in teaspoons rather than ounces, because your baby has a very small tummy the first few days after birth. Colostrum is a very high concentration of nutrition for your baby and is full of antibodies. It acts like a natural laxative to help your baby eliminate the meconium in its system. Meconium is the undigested debris from the amniotic fluid in the baby's digestive system (the poop that looks like black tar poop). It also aids baby in expelling excess bilirubin, which helps prevent newborn jaundice.

Some moms wonder if this colostrum is enough for their baby, and, indeed, it is. Keep in mind that when a baby is first born, his or her stomach is only about the size of a marble. On day three it's about the size of a shooter marble, and on day seven it's finally the size of a ping-pong ball. Usually Mom's milk comes in around day two or three, and by then most of the meconium is out of baby's system. The poop has changed from that black tar consistency to a mustard yellow color, and his or her tummy is ready for more substance.

During this time I recommend you nurse your baby as often as baby desires. Frequent feedings ensure baby is getting enough. I usually recommend every two or three hours during the day. Then at night if the baby goes longer between feedings, it's okay. Count your blessings. In the first week, you may experience some engorgement. Your body will regulate itself according to how much your baby consumes at each feeding.

When your baby was inside your womb, he or she took all the nutrients they needed first and you got any leftovers. Now that the baby is born, your body takes all the nutrients it needs first and baby gets the leftovers. So while you are breastfeeding, you need to consume an extra 500 calories to ensure baby is getting nice, rich milk full of nutrients versus skim milk.

Low levels of **essential fatty acids** may decrease or inhibit your milk supply. The basic vitality supplements offer the perfect amounts of essential omega fatty acids to help with this. If you feel your body is craving more, you can add extra omega three's to your daily routine. They have the best source for your fatty acids. Try fennel or basil essential oil to help you increase your milk supply. You can apply all over to the breast, avoiding the nipple, three or four times a day after breastfeeding. There is no need to wash it off before breast-feeding. You can also take these oils internally in a capsule or directly under your tongue and chase with water.

Another thing that has been known to increase milk production is **zinc**. Often after being sick you will notice a decrease in milk flow. This is because your body has used up all its zinc supply to get well. Taking a zinc supplement may help to increase the supply. Zinc is also found in the basic vitality supplements.

Peppermint is an oil that may decrease milk supply. I say "may" because remember, everybody is different. With some moms peppermint has no effect, and for others just smelling it will decrease their milk supply. So if you are using peppermint for a headache or fever, pay attention to your body and see how it reacts. One or two drops every now and again for a headache may be okay. Four or five drops a day may not. Again, just experiment and see how your body responds. Blends with peppermint in them are generally okay, because the peppermint is in such a small amount it doesn't usually have the same effect as the single peppermint oil, but start out slow and see how your body responds. The seasonal blend softgels are safe for pregnancy or while breastfeeding, but keep in mind they do have peppermint in them. If you notice a significant decrease in milk supply, you can make your own capsules with 2 drops each of lemon, lavender and melaleuca (replacing the peppermint with melaleuca). Metabolic blend is also safe to take while breastfeeding but keep in mind, it does have peppermint in it and peppermint may decrease your milk supply so you will want to start slow just like any other blend that contains peppermint. Also, this is not a time to diet or cut calories, you don't want to use a metabolic blend to curb your appetite while breastfeeding.

Dry or cracked nipples are common during the time right after birth. It's usually the result of an improper latch. A baby's nursing position is vital to a good latch. Make sure baby doesn't have to turn its head to nurse. Also that you have as much of the areola in baby's mouth as possible, and check to assure it's an even amount all the way around. Your baby should be belly to belly with you, and his bottom lip should be pulled out as opposed to sucked in. I recommend a cotton nursing pad instead of a disposable one, as they can cause problems like thrush and infections from the chemicals in the pads. If you do experience dry or cracked nipples, you can apply myrrh, geranium, or sandalwood directly on the affected area. You can dilute with a drop of fractionated coconut oil, but it also can be applied undiluted. Do this right after nursing, and then there is no need to wash it off before the next nursing session. You might find corrective ointment helpful. It enhances the natural process of healing. It also provides a moisture barrier that helps to protect the skin. Dr. Jack Newman at breastfeedinginc.ca has much more information than I can provide here for breastfeeding tips.

When your baby is having a growth spurt, you may feel like you are not making enough milk. Growth spurts are temporary, but to help meet the needs of your baby you may feel the need to increase your supply. Other times you may notice a decrease in milk supply is when you menstruate or ovulate, there are great essential oils that can help to **increase milk supply**. Apply two to three drops fennel in a capsule and take by mouth internally three to four times a day. Apply one to two drops basil topically on the breast, avoiding the nipple, three to four times a day. This may help increase milk supply by the next day. When you notice an increase, you can discontinue the fennel and basil. You must increase calories by 500 when breast-feeding to make enough caloric and fat filled milk for babe. Nurse as often as you can to help bring up the supply and demand.

Some women are more prone to **breast infections** than others. Moms who tend to have clogged ducts are usually milk drinkers. Try eliminating dairy from your diet. You should see a difference. Another tip is to change your nursing position often so the baby can empty all the ducts. You may notice an area that usually starts out as a hard lump that may be a little pinkish and tender. This is a clogged duct, and it can be unclogged by gently massaging it in a downward motion toward the nipple. This will usually resolve it as long as you catch it in a timely manner. However, keep in mind that it can change to a full-blown infection, sometimes as quickly as two hours. If this happens it is very painful, and the infection is accompanied by fever, body aches, and chills. You may feel like you have the flu.

I recommend taking 1000 milligrams of vitamin C every hour. Also, massage some antibiotic category oils diluted with fractionated coconut oil directly onto that area of the breast. In addition, I recommend putting three or four drops of melaleuca, thyme, clove, and oregano in a capsule and taking one every one or two hours until you notice an improvement. After that, back off to four times a day for a week, to make sure all infection is gone.

I like to use four different oils in a capsule of four drops each and rotate, using a different combination each time. One of my favorite homeopathic remedies I recommend for the occasional breast infections is phytolacca in a 30c dose. You can get it at a health food store that carries homeopathic remedies. If not, order it online. You will only need three to four pellets under your tongue two to three times a day for a day or two. It works like magic.

Breastfeeding Tips

- Drink three to four quarts of water daily.
- Don't drink milk.
- Take extra zinc.
- Use anti-stress/relaxation oils.
- Basic nutrient trio supplements daily

Babies respond to FLOW, when they have to work for the milk they loose interest and get frustrated.

Occasionally, for various reasons, you may need to decrease your milk supply. Try two or three drops of peppermint essential oil in a capsule or a warm tea internally three to five times a day to **decrease milk supply**. Regular peppermint tea will not have much effect on it, but just one drop of peppermint essential oils is twenty-eight times stronger than one cup of regular peppermint tea.

If you feel **engorged** or your breasts are too full, you may want to express just enough milk to relieve the fullness. Sometimes even a warm shower is enough for you to be comfortable. If you express too much, your body will assume it needs to make more. The less milk you release, the more quickly your body will figure out that it needs to decrease its production. Your grandma might tell you to bind your breasts to dry up, but this may cause plugged ducts and can lead to breast infections or abscess.

Newborns

*O*ne of my favorite parts of being at a birth is putting frankincense on a babe in the first hours after he or she is born. Many cultures do this as a religious practice. I personally think it reduces stress and aids in the bonding experience between parents and babe. When a baby is born, that child comes into a world that is very new. As intense as this experience was for Mom, think about how intense it was for babe. I can't think of any better essential oil than a drop of frankincense on the baby's crown and down the spine to help baby feel that everything's going to be okay.

I love lavender and the calming blend. Both of these can be used with fractionated coconut oil as an excellent carrier oil to use on your baby with great results. You can also diffuse a drop or two of Roman chamomile in your baby's room to help relieve tummy discomfort or support a restful nights sleep.

An abstract in the journal *Early Human Development* cites a study in which infants were given a bath, some with and some without lavender-scented bath oil. The mothers in the lavender bath oil group were more relaxed. They smiled and touched their infants more during the bath. Their infants looked at them a greater percentage of the bath time, cried less, and spent more time in a deep sleep after the bath. The cortisol levels of this group of mothers and infants significantly decreased. This confirmed the behavioral data showing increased relaxation of the mothers and their infants.

These findings support a body of research regarding the relaxing and sleep-inducing properties of lavender aroma. High quality, pure lavender is the way to go when dealing with a baby. Make sure that the lavender you use is a high quality, independently tested therapeutic grade.

The umbilical cord has served for nine months as the method by which babe has been nourished. When the cord is cut, it is an open line to every system in the baby's body. I have found that myrrh is helpful in creating a liquid seal on this site to protect all systems of the body. I put one drop undiluted on and around the cord stump.

I love grounding blend on baby's feet. Babies have come from their home (the womb) that they have known for nine months. They have been snuggled in warm water with all their needs met. And now they have been through this stressful birth experience of being squished through this strange canal, and into a bright, cold, unfamiliar world. Sometimes I think babes want to go back inside. This is where grounding blend comes in handy. It helps baby remember, oh yes, I think I am supposed to be here, and these voices sound familiar. I think I might stay. One drop of grounding blend can be applied undiluted to the bottoms of baby's feet.

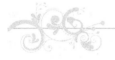

"Stephanie massaged frankincense, grounding blend, and myrrh essential oils on my baby within minutes of her being born. My sweet baby girl was calm and had no respiratory issues. She nursed successfully within the first few minutes."

—Ashley in Utah

Melissa is one of the most powerful essential oils we have in helping us remember our original blueprint and in aiding us to reach our greatest and highest potential. It raises our body's vibration and reminds us of our spiritual contacts. It repairs DNA damage from thoughts, emotions, and other negative experiences we may have had inside the womb and through the birthing process. It helps us be in harmony with our true spirit, enabling us to let go of any negativity that does not uniquely belong to each of us personally.

Moms may have had thoughts of, *How am I going to afford this baby?* or, *This baby came at the worst time for me!* or even thoughts of wishing it were the other gender. These thoughts may be resolved by birth as far as the parents go, but babies know! They felt that feeling at the time of that thought's conception. Babies are affected by that energy and the feelings that accompany it. Melissa helps to repair any self-doubt and disharmonious energy. We all have negative thoughts at one time or another. Certainly they are not meant to bring disharmony to your baby in the womb on purpose, but it happens anyway. Melissa comes to the rescue to offer the divine love and the joy of being here. Every mother and baby needs Melissa every day!

Oils for baby after birth

- **Frankincense:** Apply one drop undiluted on the crown of head and spine as protection and bonding. It also assists in circulation and transfer of oxygen in the cells.

- **Myrrh:** Apply one drop undiluted on the umbilical cord to help seal the tissue and protect all systems of the body.

- **Grounding blend:** Apply one drop undiluted on feet to ground and align the babe.

- **Melissa:** Apply a scant drop undiluted on bottoms of feet for DNA repair.

"I have continued to use the grounding blend and frankincense on Micah David almost every day since he was born. We have gotten so many compliments on how calm, alert, mature, and happy our little boy is. I know without doubt that the use of essential oils

can be credited in giving him the healthiest start in life."

—Jenny in Arizona

"I loved, loved, loved using essential oils before, during, and after my pregnancy! It was by far the best pregnancy I have had. I used them with my third baby. I used lemon or any other citrus oil in all my water, and I never experienced swelling. I took the basic vitality supplements, and I feel my hormones were always balanced.

"I rubbed frankincense and lavender on my abdomen every day to reduce stretch marks. When anti-aging blend came out, I switched and used that every day. I loved knowing that as a mom I could help my baby have the best 'in-house' experience.

"My recovery was so quick that I had to remind myself when I got tired that I'd just had a baby. The anti-aging blend made healing a very quick process.

"I loved having the oils for after delivery to continue to help baby 'out of house.' Because I used

grounding blend, frankincense, Melissa, protective blend, digestive blend, and respiratory blend oils in a daily regimen, my baby was six months old before he ever got sick. He went through flu season, RSV season, traveled all over the United States, and had been around a lot of people. I know he was protected because he was in his own essential oil bubble."

—Kathy in Utah

Well Baby Care

*P*ut frankincense on your baby's back and grounding blend on his feet every day to balance all body systems. These work great mixed with a natural hand and body lotion or fractionated coconut oil as a daily massage instead of traditional baby lotion.

"My two-year-old son had febrile seizures for three months straight. I started putting frankincense on him daily. I put it up and down his spine, as well as

on the three triangle spots behind each ear and at the base of his neck. It has now almost been a year of no seizures!"

—Jamie in Arizona

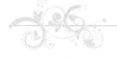

You will commonly see the baby's tongue coated with a milk-like substance. This is called **thrush**. Your baby may even have a diaper rash that can turn very red and raw quickly. Thrush is a yeast infection, and it can spread to mom's nipple as well. You will want to treat both baby's mouth and your nipple so you avoid passing it back and forth to each other. Put a few drops of melaleuca directly on affected areas, both the nipple and baby's mouth, undiluted or diluted with fraction-ated coconut oil. Mom should pay attention to her diet and make sure she has cut out all refined sugar and simple carbohydrates. Dairy may contribute to yeast also.

Sixty percent of all babies get a mild form of **jaundice**. This usually peaks around day three as the liver is trying to break up the bilirubin in the body. Use one drop on the bottom of baby's feet at every diaper change of geranium, lemon, or rosemary to help support the liver in breaking up the bilirubin. Indirect sunlight also helps break up the bilirubin into smaller particles. Undress baby to expose as much skin as possible, and sit with babe in some indirect sunlight a few times a day.

Usually **colic or tummy aches** point back to Mom's diet. The first thing I would recommend is Mom cutting from her diet all dairy products. This might seem hard, but if you think about the pain your baby is experiencing, it should be an easy thing to do. If your baby cries for no known reason and pulls its legs up, has a tight belly, or has a cry like he is in pain, digestive blend or fennel on baby's tummy mixed with fractionated coconut oil, or even a scant drop applied undiluted, will be your friend.

Rubbing a drop of melaleuca and basil around baby's ear may help alleviate pain from **ear discomfort**. Remember to reapply. Don't think that one time will always take care of this or any issue. The key is to reapply as often as needed, and the blessing is you CAN reapply as often as needed for pain. No need to wait four to six hours as suggested on traditional over-the-counter medications.

"My toddler was up all night crying. I didn't know what was wrong until morning when he told me repeatedly that his ear hurt. This was his first ear infection. I rubbed basil and melaleuca all around his ears. The leftover on my finger I wiped right inside his ear. Within that hour he was relieved enough to fall asleep. I put a couple drops of both melaleuca and basil on a cotton ball and put the cotton in his ear while he slept. He took a three-hour nap, and when he

woke up, he no longer complained about his ear! Less than three hours and his ear infection was better!"

—Jamie in Arizona

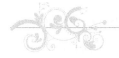

For **diaper rash**, use sandalwood or myrrh in fractionated coconut oil and lightly coat the area. You may also use anti-aging blend, lavender, helichrysum, or melaleuca.

For pain while your child is **teething**, apply two drops of white fir directly to the gums, or add one drop of clove to one tablespoon of fractionated coconut oil and apply to the gums. Melaleuca and Roman chamomile both work well, too.

For an alternative to **baby powder**, add twenty drops of lavender to eight tablespoons of cornstarch.

The best thing you can do for an **eye infection** or any goopy eye issue is to squirt a little breast milk directly into baby's eye. The white blood cells and antibodies in the breast milk will clear up any infection fairly quickly. Always use fresh milk; you may need to express some in a cup and use an eyedropper to drop it directly into your baby's eye. You may also have success with lavender diluted with a drop of fractionated coconut oil; pat it around the eye bone.

A **fever** is the body's way of recognizing there is something wrong going on. The body is trying to get rid of it. The fever itself is not bad. It's the way you feel when you have a fever that is not so fun. Just one drop of peppermint on the bottoms of your baby's feet will generally resolve a fever quickly. Patchouli is another great oil to help with fevers. This can be applied every fifteen to thirty minutes as needed to the bottom of the feet.

Circumcision is a medical procedure done on newborn baby boys. I recommend the same peri spray for the circumcision site as I recommend for a new mom. Lavender and frankincense is a great combination for soothing and aiding in the healing of this raw area. Mix equal parts of frankincense, lavender, and fractionated coconut oil in an empty oil bottle and put a spray top on it. Use at every diaper change.

To alleviate **dry skin**, a mix of frankincense and fractionated coconut oil is a great mix for a baby massage. Lavender or calming blend is a good choice for a massage at night to help relax baby and start a routine for bedtime. Try a natural hand and body lotion, a great unscented lotion for hydrating dry skin, and add the therapeutic oil of your choice.

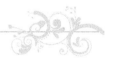

"I use protective blend on Aiva's feet morning and night to help support her immune system! She gets an oil rubdown with calming blend, lavender, digestive blend, respiratory blend, joyful blend, and coconut oil every night after a bath!"

—Phalecia in Utah

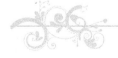

Postpartum Depression

*P*ostpartum depression affects ten to fifteen percent of all new moms. There are many changes that are happening in Mom's body, both physically and emotionally. Hormonal changes can cause stress to the entire body. After the baby is born and the newness wears off, everyone's life returns to normal, except Mom's. Hers will never be the same. She may be overwhelmed with the responsibility of caring for this new babe, in addition to the already existing responsibilities she has. Sometimes the realization of this can be over-whelming and result in the "baby blues" or full-on depression.

The basic vitality supplements taken every day can help balance hormones quickly and help Mom have more energy and feel less stressed as she cares for her new baby and comes into balance with a new normal in her life. The most common nutritional defi-ciencies in those who suffer from depressive disorders are B vitamins, omega 3, and magnesium. These are all included in the basic vitality supplements in the perfect amounts.

Essential oils that will support and uplift you in this changing time are any of the following: grounding blend, calming blend, joyful blend, women's monthly blend, bergamot, wild orange, clary sage, cypress, frankincense, geranium, lavender, Roman chamomile, rosewood, sandalwood, or blend for women. I recom-mend using any of these as a personal perfume that you wear daily. Not only will you smell great, you'll be uplifting your emotions at the same time.

Do not underestimate the power of citrus oils. They help normalize neuroendocrine hormone levels and immune function. Basil helps neurotransmitters, and lavender stimulates serotonin release. There are so many choices to assist you with postpartum changes.

Diffusing is another great way to get these oils into your system, along with taking them internally. Frankincense is a great oil to help with any kind of depression. I recommend taking four or five drops under your tongue and chasing with water every day, or you may also put the oil in a capsule.

Every day gives us different experiences and emotions. While each essential oil is similar, they all have their own individual strengths and purposes to include supporting us emotionally. These oils blends are specifically formulated to help us through the times when our emotions are in need of TLC:

- Encouraging Blend contains mint and citrus oils known to energize and elevate

- Uplifting Blend contains citrus and spice oils known to excite and intrigue

- Inspiring Blend contains spice and herb/grass oils known to sooth and attract

- Renewing Blend contains herb/grass and tree oils known to balance and clarify

- Comforting Blend contains tree and floral oils known to comfort and ground

- Reassuring Blend contains floral and mint oils known to calm and support

To use the essential oils when supporting emotions, you can diffuse aromatically or you can apply 1–2 drops in your palms, rub hands together, and inhale deeply from hands. You can also apply topically to touch points such as the back of the neck, wrists, and over the heart.

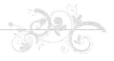

"I used grounding blend for emotional and postpartum support after I delivered my second child. I felt its calming and grounding effect every day."

—Christine in Arizona

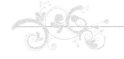

Postpartum Depression Blends

Any of the following blends would work great as room diffusers or in a room mister or spray. You can also use them topically as lotions, or place a drop on a pillowcase at bedtime or in a warm bath with sea salt.

Blend 1

- 1 drop rose
- 1 drop wild orange
- 3 drops sandalwood

Blend 2

- 1 drop lavender
- 3 drops grapefruit
- 1 drop ylang ylang

Blend 3

- 1 drop bergamot
- 1 drop grapefruit
- 1 drop clary sage
- 1 drop wild orange
- 3 drops frankincense

Miscarriage

$\mathcal{W}$hen someone miscarries, it is one of the most heartbreaking emotions for both parents. There is always a feeling of helplessness and the question, "What did I do wrong?" Who or what is to blame? In the case of a threatening miscarriage, there's always the question whether or not to do anything or just let nature takes its course. My philosophy is that the body needs support, and a great way to do that is by using the grounding blend. Either there's something wrong and your body is trying to abort, or it just needs a little more assistance to sustain a healthy pregnancy. Using both basic vitality supplements and the essential oils will help support your body's natural balance and help it do whatever is best.

If you are experiencing menstrual-type cramping and you are worried about a possible miscarriage, my suggestion is to put five or six drops each of myrrh and frankincense into a capsule and insert it vaginally, high into the cervix, at night. Do this each night until the concern has passed. Roman chamomile topically may help relax the uterus if you are experiencing contractions. Frankincense and lavender may be applied topically to abdomen as stabilizers.

The uterus is a muscle, and often intercourse will bring on contractions because of the release of prostaglandins. Roman chamomile, frankincense, and lavender massaged on the lower belly may help relax the uterus so it stops contracting. Think about the oils that help with relaxation; these are the oils of choice when you want to stop contractions.

Once you know that a miscarriage is definitely the path your body is taking, then clary sage may help support your body through this big undertaking.

A note here about clary sage: Some might ask, "Should I avoid clary sage during pregnancy if it brings on contractions?" My answer is that there is no need to avoid it if your body isn't contracting. Clary sage is in the women's monthly blend, which is great for hormone support before, during, and after pregnancy. Women in general experience an overall hormonal balance when they use women's monthly blend during pregnancy. If I had a client who was having preterm labor, I would recommend women's monthly blend, but I wouldn't recommend clary sage by itself. Women's monthly blend is going to be more balancing, and clary sage used separately may make contractions that are already happening a little stronger.

Think of going into a room where there is soft lighting, everything is lit up, and you can see fine, nothing is harsh or too strong. You could even look directly at that light and feel comfortable with that gentle light.

This is how women's monthly blend works in our body, it is very gentle and calming, but perfect to support and balance our hormones in pregnancy in a very gentle way.

Now imaging going into a room where the light is extremely bright, it is almost too bright for your eyes to look at directly. This is how clary sage is, it is like a very strong, bright light. It is great to zone in on your hormones when you need it, but in pregnancy, we are looking for balance, not change.

This is why I teach that clary sage "may" help strengthen contractions once they have started, because it's zoning in on the contraction. Keep in mind it will not bring them on unless everything is already in perfect alignment for labor.

I usually recommend avoiding clary sage in pregnancy until 40 weeks, then in labor, if you need to intensify or strengthen contractions clary sage is perfect. This is not going to force the body to go beyond what it's capable of. It's adaptogenic and very supportive in labor.

- Apply clary sage to lower abdominal area to promote uterine contractions and assist in passing remaining tissue.

- Apply soothing blend or a combination of lavender and white fir to abdomen for pain relief.

- Continue applying layers on abdomen or bottoms of the feet clary sage, geranium, and lavender to balance both physical and emotional needs.

Remember to address your emotional well-being with morning and evening application of blends such as grounding blend, joyful blend, and calming blend, encouraging blend, uplifting blend, inspiring blend, renewing blend, comforting blend, reassuring blend, or single oils such as frankincense and wild orange or sandalwood and invigorating blend.

Miscarriage Grief Blend

- 3 drop elevation
- 4 drops bergamot
- 8 drops cypress
- 8 drops frankincense
- Diffuse or put a couple of drops in hands inhale and apply to back of neck and around ears

Everyday Routine

*P*reventative health care means continuing a daily habit so you don't have to remember the details while caring for you and your newborn! Establish a daily routine for you and your baby for optimal health. Don't wait until you get sick or are stressed to use them. Preventative is the key.

Following are everyday oils you can place under your tongue. This is my personal preference because I don't like to take the time to make capsules, but if you wish, you can make capsules with your everyday oils.

Or simply put the oils on the bottoms of your feet or on the back of your neck. I think they hold great value in taking them internally, but the most important thing is just using them, whichever way works best for you.

- Apply grounding blend and protective blend to feet every morning.
- 1 drop Melissa under the tongue every morning.
- 3 to 5 drops of frankincense under the tongue every morning.
- 10 drops of grapefruit in a capsule or under the tongue.
- Metabolic blend: 3 to 5 drops, three to five times a day (use caution while breastfeeding), or 3 to 5 gel caps a day.
- Detoxification blend (optional): 3 to 5 drops in capsule, or topically on liver area, or 1 to 2 gel caps a day.
- Lemon in ALL your water. Drinking three to four quarts daily.
- Basic vitality supplements (the BEST prenatal vitamin).

- Take probiotic defense formula daily. Take 1 to 2 daily.
- Digestive enzyme complex: Take 1 upon waking, 1 at bedtime, and 1 to 2 with every meal.
- Apply to feet before bed a few drops of favorite stress-free oils: Roman chamomile, bergamot, frankincense, lavender, calming blend, and vetiver.

Pregnancy and Birth Kit Suggestions

- **Basil:** Soothes sore muscles and joints. Assists with clear breathing. Acts as a cooling agent for the skin. Soothes minor skin irritations. Apply to breast to increase milk supply. Promotes mental alertness. Enhances memory function. Sharpens focus while studying or reading. Lessens anxious feelings. Reduces stress. Reduces tension when applied to temples and back of neck.

☙ **Cypress:** Assists with circulation and clear breathing. Promotes healthy respiratory function. Soothes tight, tense muscles. Supports localized blood flow. Beneficial for oily skin conditions.

☙ **Digestive Blend:** Aids in digestion. Eases occasional stomach discomfort. Supports a healthy gastrointestinal track.

☙ **Frankincense:** Helps build and maintain a healthy immune system. Promotes cellular health. Reduces the appearance of blemishes and rejuvenates skin. Promotes feelings of peace, relaxation, satisfaction, and overall wellness. Good to apply to baby's crown and back at birth.

☙ **Grapefruit:** Ten to fifteen drops in a capsule daily to support cortisol/stress levels. Cleanses and purifies. Supports healthy metabolism. Helps reduce mental and physical fatigue. Helps with sore muscles and joints.

- **Geranium:** Promotes clear, healthy skin. Helps calm nerves and lessen stress. Supports liver health. Apply to baby's feet to help support liver in breaking up bilirubin.

- **Ginger:** Helps ease occasional indigestion and nausea. Promotes overall digestive health.

- **Grounding Blend:** Enhances effects of other oils. Creates a sense of calm and well-being. Promotes whole-body relaxation. Brings harmony to the mind and body. Evokes feelings of tranquility and balance. Promotes circulation. Supports cellular health and overall well-being. Lessens stress and helps with anxious feelings and nerves. Apply to baby's feet at birth. Good to use EVERY DAY.

- **Helichrysum:** Used as tissue support as baby is crowning. Helps skin recover quickly. Promotes healthy liver function. Supports localized blood flow. Helps detoxify the body. Promotes circulation. Helps reduce the

appearance of wrinkles and other blemishes.
Promotes a glowing, youthful complexion.
Helps relieve tension.

- **Invigorating Blend:** Combination of all
citrus oils to support your immune system.
Cleanses and purifies air and surfaces. Helps
reduce stress and uplifts mood. Positively
affects mood with energizing and refreshing
properties.

- **Lavender:** Supports blocked tear ducts.
Widely used for its calming and relaxing qualities. Soothes occasional skin irritations. Helps
skin recover quickly. Eases muscle tension.

- **Lemon:** Cleanses and purifies the air and surfaces. Naturally cleanses the body and aids in
digestion. Supports healthy respiratory function. Promotes a positive mood and cognitive
ability. Helps ward off free radicals with its
antioxidant benefits. Soothes an irritated

throat. Supports baby to process bilirubin at birth.

- **Melaleuca:** Renowned for its cleansing and rejuvenating effect on the skin. Promotes healthy immune function. Protects against environmental and seasonal threats. Promotes a clear, healthy complexion. Soothes minor skin irritations. Helps purify and freshen the air.

- **Myrrh:** Powerful cleansing properties, especially for the mouth and throat. Soothes the skin. Promotes emotional balance and well-being. Apply to baby's umbilicus after cord is clamped and cut to help cord dry quickly and seal the opening. May help to support the optimal fetal position.

- **Peppermint:** Promotes healthy respiratory function and clear breathing. Alleviates occasional stomach upset. May help to support the optimal fetal position.

- **Protective Blend:** USE DAILY to support healthy immune function. Protects against environmental threats. Cleans surfaces. Purifies the skin while promoting healthy circulation. Energizing, uplifting aroma.

- **Soothing Blend or Tension Blend:** Eases muscle tension in the head and neck. Helps reduce tension, stress, and worry. Soothes the mind and body. Calms emotions.

- **Wild Orange:** Powerful cleanser and purifying agent. Protects against seasonal and environmental threats. Uplifting to the mind and body. Supports baby to process bilirubin at birth.

- **Women's Monthly Blend:** Helps balance hormones. Provides temporary respite from cramps, hot flashes, and emotional swings.

- **Fractionated Coconut Oil:** Carrier or diluting oil.

Basic Midwife Kit

- **Clary Sage:** May increase strength of contractions once labor starts. Soothes discomfort associated with menstrual cycles. Helps balance hormones. Soothes nervous tension and lightens mood. Calming and soothing to the skin.

- **Frankincense:** Helps build and maintain a healthy immune system. Promotes cellular health. Reduces the appearance of blemishes and rejuvenates skin. Promotes feelings of peace, relaxation, satisfaction, and overall wellness. Good to apply to baby's crown and back at birth.

☙ **Grounding Blend:** Enhances effects of other oils. Creates a sense of calm and well-being. Promotes whole-body relaxation. Brings harmony to the mind and body. Evokes feelings of tranquility and balance. Promotes circulation. Supports cellular health and overall well-being. Lessens stress and helps with anxious feelings and nerves. Apply to baby's feet at birth. Good to use EVERY DAY.

☙ **Helichrysum:** Used as tissue support as baby is crowning. Helps skin recover quickly. Promotes healthy liver function. Supports localized blood flow. Helps detoxify the body. Promotes circulation. Helps reduce the appearance of wrinkles and other blemishes. Promotes a glowing, youthful complexion. Helps relieve tension.

- **Lavender:** Supports blocked tear ducts. Widely used for its calming and relaxing qualities. Soothes occasional skin irritations. Helps skin recover quickly. Eases muscle tension.

- **Lemon:** Cleanses and purifies the air and surfaces. Naturally cleanses the body and aids in digestion. Supports healthy respiratory function. Promotes a positive mood and cognitive ability. Helps ward off free radicals with its antioxidant benefits. Soothes an irritated throat. Supports baby to process bilirubin at birth.

- **Myrrh:** Powerful cleansing properties, especially for the mouth and throat. Soothes the skin. Promotes emotional balance and well-being. Apply to baby's umbilicus after cord is clamped and cut to help cord dry quickly and seal the opening. May help to support the optimal fetal position.

- **Peppermint:** Promotes healthy respiratory function and clear breathing. Alleviates occasional stomach upset. May help to support the optimal fetal position.

- **Soothing Blend Rub:** Eases muscle tension in the head and neck. Helps reduce stress and worry. Soothes the mind and body. Calms emotions.

- **White Fir:** Provides soothing support to sore muscles and joints. Supports clear breathing and respiratory function. Energizes the body and the mind. Evokes feelings of stability, energy, and empowerment. Helps the body relax.

- **Wild Orange:** Powerful cleanser and purifying agent. Protects against seasonal and environmental threats. Uplifting to the mind and body. Supports baby to process bilirubin at birth.

- **Fractionated Coconut Oil:** Carrier or diluting oil.

Essential Midwife Kit

- **Anti-aging Blend:** Reduces the appearance of fine lines and wrinkles. Helps reduce contributing factors to aging skin. Supports skin at a cellular level. Helps sustain smoother, more radiant, and youthful skin. Supports the normal stretch marks in pregnancy. Promotes tissue repair. Used for postpartum peri spray.

- **Basil:** Soothes sore muscles and joints. Assists with clear breathing. Acts as a cooling agent for the skin. Soothes minor skin irritations.

Apply to breast to increase milk supply. Promotes mental alertness. Enhances memory function. Sharpens focus while studying or reading. Lessens anxious feelings. Reduces stress. Reduces tension when applied to temples and back of neck.

- **Black Pepper:** Supports occasional back labor. Rich source of antioxidants. Supports healthy circulation. Aids digestion. Enhances food flavor. Helps ward off environmental and seasonal threats. Soothes nerves and lessens anxious feelings.

- **Clary Sage:** May increase strength of contractions once labor starts. Soothes discomfort associated with menstrual cycles. Helps balance hormones. Soothes nervous tension and lightens mood. Calming and soothing to the skin.

- **Fennel:** Relieves occasional indigestion and digestive troubles. Eases menstrual cycles.

Supports a healthy lymphatic system. Calms minor skin irritation. Apply topically to breasts to increase milk supply.

- **Frankincense:** Helps build and maintain a healthy immune system. Promotes cellular health. Reduces the appearance of blemishes and rejuvenates skin. Promotes feelings of peace, relaxation, satisfaction, and overall wellness. Good to apply to baby's crown and back at birth.

- **Geranium:** Promotes clear, healthy skin. Helps calm nerves and lessen stress. Supports liver health. Apply to baby's feet to help support liver in breaking up bilirubin.

- **Grounding Blend:** Enhances effects of other oils. Creates a sense of calm and well-being. Promotes whole-body relaxation. Brings harmony to the mind and body. Evokes feelings of tranquility and balance. Promotes circulation. Supports cellular health and overall well-being. Lessens stress and helps with anxious feelings and nerves. Apply to baby's feet at birth. Good to use EVERY DAY.

- **Helichrysum:** Used as tissue support as baby is crowning. Helps skin recover quickly. Promotes healthy liver function. Supports localized blood flow. Helps detoxify the body. Promotes circulation. Helps reduce the appearance of wrinkles and other blemishes. Promotes a glowing, youthful complexion. Helps relieve tension.

- **Lavender:** Supports blocked tear ducts. Widely used for its calming and relaxing qualities. Soothes occasional skin irritations. Helps skin recover quickly. Eases muscle tension.

- **Lemon:** Cleanses and purifies the air and surfaces. Naturally cleanses the body and aids in digestion. Supports healthy respiratory function. Promotes a positive mood and cognitive ability. Helps ward off free radicals with its antioxidant benefits. Soothes an irritated throat. Supports baby to process bilirubin at birth.

Massage Blend: Relaxes muscles and soothes joints. Promotes circulation. Helps to calm and soothe target areas.

Melissa: Supports healthy DNA. Supports the body in its perfect blueprint. Helps boost a healthy immune system. Calms tension and nerves. Addresses occasional stomach discomfort. Helps initiate a restful sleep. Promotes emotional and cognitive health.

Myrrh: Powerful cleansing properties, especially for the mouth and throat. Soothes the skin. Promotes emotional balance and well-being. Apply to baby's umbilicus after cord is clamped and cut to help cord dry quickly and seal the opening. May help to support the optimal fetal position.

- **Peppermint:** Promotes healthy respiratory function and clear breathing. Alleviates occasional stomach upset. May help to support the optimal fetal position.

- **Soothing Blend Rub:** Eases muscle tension in the head and neck. Helps reduce stress and worry. Soothes the mind and body. Calms emotions.

- **White Fir:** Provides soothing support to sore muscles and joints. Supports clear breathing and respiratory function. Energizes the body and the mind. Evokes feelings of stability, energy, and empowerment. Helps the body relax.

- **Wild Orange:** Powerful cleanser and purifying agent. Protects against seasonal and environmental threats. Uplifting to the mind and body. Supports baby to process bilirubin at birth.

- **Women's Monthly Blend:** Helps balance hormones. Provides temporary respite from cramps, hot flashes, and emotional swings.

- **Fractionated Coconut Oil:** Carrier or diluting oil.

Premium Midwife Kit

Every oil!

Sources

- *The Complete Book of Essential Oils &
  Aromatherapy* by Valerie Ann Worwood

- *A Guide to Motherhood* by Katherine Tarr

- *The Encyclopedia of Aromatherapy* by Chrissie
  Wildwood

- *Emotional Healing with Essential Oils* by Daniel
  Macdonald

- *Midwifery Today* Numbers 69 and 79

About the Author

Stephanie Fritz, also known as The Essential Midwife, has a very successful midwifery practice in Southeast Arizona. She covers an area 2.5 hours all around her from the desert to the mountains. Many of her 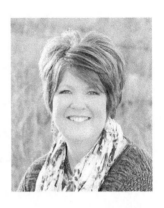 out-of-hospital births are in very rural areas. She is the mother of four daughters, three of which were born at home, and all breastfed. These experiences have shaped her vision of what women's health care should be. She knows first-hand what a difference information and a sense of control can make when having a baby.

She believes that knowledge is power. With comfort, support, trust and privacy, birth can be simple and beautiful. She loves to empower the families she serves through education and choices, by teaching them that as they take their health into their own hands they can improve their lives.

She believes the relationship with her clients is very important, and can have a strong impact on the birth. She often says her clients are her best friends. She offers in depth and personal prenatal visits where care is given to the mother's emotional needs as well as the normal physical assessment of mother's and baby's well-being. It is important to feel comfortable, as this is the time to bond and create trusting relationships. Her clients will tell you she has a special gift to always make you feel better when you leave than when you came. It's not uncommon for tears and laughter to be shared in the same hour.

She has enjoyed using essential oils since the 80"s with her family and has experienced the many benefits they offer. Over the last several years the quality and purity of essential oils has improved and far surpassed anything she has used in the past. In 2008 she was introduced to a quality of therapeutic essential oils that she felt confident in using with her clients and their babies as a natural health solution. She has watched her clients' health and comfort increase dramatically in the last eight years both physically as well as emotionally with these gifts of the earth.

She loves to share how these powerful plant extracts can empower you whether you are a midwife, doula, mom or just someone who wants to take control of your health in a natural way.

"Essential oils are one of the most powerful tools I have in helping to keep the family's I serve happy and healthy. I know these essential oils have helped my clients have an easier pregnancy, labor and postpartum as well as ease my job as their midwife".

Essential oils have the potential to enhance and compliment every woman's right to a fabulous pregnancy, labor and birth experience.

Stephanie is a Licensed Midwife (LM) and Certified Professional Midwife (CPM), a Therapeutic Gemstone Practitioner, Author, Public Speaker, Essential Oil Educator and an AromaTherapy Technique Trainer.

Index